黃帝內經素問:陰陽應象大論

HUÁNG DÌ NÈI JĪNG SÙ WÈN:
YĪN YÁNG YÌNG XIÀNG DÀ LÙN

HUMMING WITH ELEPHANTS THE GREAT TREATISE ON THE RESONANT MANIFESTATIONS OF YĪN AND YÁNG

A TRANSLATION AND DISCUSSION OF THE
YELLOW EMPEROR'S INNER CLASSIC
PLAIN QUESTIONS CHAPTER 5

ALSO BY SABINE WILMS

The Divine Farmer's Classic of Materia Medica
神農本草經 *Shén Nóng Běncǎo Jīng*

Twelve Characters:
A Transmission of Wang Fengyi's Teachings

Let the Radiant Yang Shine Forth:
Lectures on Virtue by Liu Yousheng

Venerating the Root:
Sun Simiao's *Bei Ji Qian Jin Yao Fang,*
Volume 5 on Pediatrics • Parts One and Two

黄帝內經素問:陰陽應象大論

Huáng Dì Nèi Jīng Sù Wèn: Yīn Yáng Yìng Xiàng Dà Lùn

A Translation and Discussion of Chapter Five of the Yellow Emperor's Inner Classic Plain Questions

Humming *with* Elephants

The Great Treatise on the Resonant Manifestations of Yīn and Yáng

Sabine Wilms, PhD

HAPPY GOAT PRODUCTIONS
WHIDBEY ISLAND WA • USA

Published in the United States of America

ISBN 978-1-7321571-0-1

Cover art by © Remee L. Gemo — www.remee.gallery
Bright Circle/insert: **Autumn Leaves**, encaustic on birch, 2017

Interior photographs by © Keith Schreiber — jkschreiber.wordpress.com
Interior paintings by © Sunjae Lee — www.fermatawellness.com/paintings

Additional interior photography and illustration: Double-happy Safety Matches by DHSAM via Wikimedia Commons, Sabine Wilms, Momo Wilms-Crowe. Water cycle illustration: https://pubs.usgs.gov/wsp/2220/report.pdf.

Book design and production by Barbara Tada — www.pixelgardendesign.com

Published by Happy Goat Productions
Whidbey Island, WA • USA

For more information and to purchase
other works by Sabine Wilms, visit our website:
www.HappyGoatProductions.com

Dedication

To all healers (and yes, that includes YOU, dear reader, because that is all of our nature as humans).

To my favorite human: my beautiful, passionate, courageous daughter Momo who is determined to find her own way of healing the world by harmonizing Heaven and Earth.

To the Nagas of Whidbey Island who have awakened the mermaid in me and whose calls for a daily swim in the sea carried me across the finish line.

To all my relations, who sustain me and are sustained by me.

Contents

Foreword

THE PRACTICE OF 醫學 *YI XUE*/MEDICINE IN CHINA, CONSTANT SINCE the era of the素問 *Sù Wèn*, is an unbroken chain. Medicine, to the Chinese, is more than 'life science', it is also a philosophy of life, and a daily discipline to maintain health. It needs creativity and poetry, to inspire, to uplift.

醫 *Yi*/medicine must be based on 理 *li*/principle, an understanding of the universal laws of change codified in the 易經 *Yi jing*/Classic of Change. It must resonate with the laws of heaven and earth, to apply to all life, and remind humanity of its place in the universal scheme. Medicine is meditation on ecology.

As a 大論 *da lun*/"Great Treatise", *Sù Wèn* Chapter 5 is of extreme importance to study. It is a cognitive map that expresses the essential principles of medicine for generations to come, never to be forgotten, so that medicine can continue to exist and thrive. As a central chapter in the *Sù Wèn*, it expressed the beginning, the unifying thread, the warp, weft, and summation of 醫 *Yi*/ medicine.

As Zhang Jing-yue (Jie-bin) states in his 類經 *Lei jing*/Categorized Classic, "if you fell a tree and pull out its taproot, of the thousand branches and ten thousand leaves, none are able to survive independently." Without the taproot, the tree dies. Conversely, to remove a disease, one must extricate the taproot, so that the disease cannot return.

Without the *Sù Wèn*, Chinese and other Asian medical systems are reduced to facsimiles of their former selves. Without their root, the branches and leaves, in other words, the different schools, currents and branches of medicine cannot survive. Fine needles are inserted into human tissue, but the original intent and framework are lost.

The *Sù Wèn* is a text that benefits from multiple translations, and multiple commentaries. Sabine Wilms, one of our finest translators and teachers of the 內經 *Nei Jing* and Chinese classical medical literature, has uncovered subtle meanings in *Sù Wèn* Chapter 5, and chosen commentaries from great physicians and medical sages, such as Zhang Jingyue and Zhang Zhicong, to illuminate and freshen the original text. This little book should be a constant companion to 醫生 *yi sheng*/physicians of Chinese/Asian medicine. It is a gift to our ancient but young (in the West) profession. Read and recite its pages again and again, as within its words you will find both an anchor and a guide for your practice, an inspiration for yourself and your patients, and most important, a compass for your daily life.

Zev Rosenberg, L. Ac., 醫生 *yi sheng*
Professor, Alembic Institute
San Diego, California
Spring 2017

Introduction

"Humility in its largest sense is the knowledge of the true human position in the cosmic scale."

—Ichazo, cited in Sandra Maitri, *The Enneagrams of Passions and Virtues*

"The translator of Homer should above all be penetrated by a sense of four qualities ... that he is eminently rapid; that he is eminently plain and direct both in the evolution of his thought and in the expression of it, that is, both in his syntax and in his words; that he is eminently plain and direct in the substance of his thought, that is, in his matter and ideas; and, finally, that he is eminently noble."

—Matthew Arnold, *On Translating Homer,* as quoted by Emily Wilson in *The First Woman to Translate the Odyssey into English*[1]

The message in this book is not just about medicine for humans.
It IS Medicine for Heaven and Earth.

—The Nagas of Whidbey Island

The *Great Treatise on the Resonant Manifestations of Yīn and Yáng* (*Yīn Yáng Yìng Xiàng Dà Lùn* 陰陽應象大論, below abbreviated as *Great Treatise*) is one of the most foundational and important texts in the entire canon of Chinese medical literature. In Chinese medicine

[1] Wyatt Mason, New York Times, Nov. 2, 2017.

circles, it is also, much more prosaically and perhaps affectionately, known as *Plain Questions* Chapter Five or, even shorter, *Sù Wèn* 5. As such, it is merely a humble chapter in the "Plain Questions" (*Sù Wèn* 素問) half of the *Huáng Dì Nèi Jīng* 黃帝內經 (Inner Classic of the Yellow Emperor aka *Nèijīng*), a large collection of medical texts that was compiled in the Hàn dynasty (206 BCE to 220 CE) but contains many older layers. After having translated, worked with, and taught the *Great Treatise* to students of Chinese medicine for several years, I realized that this text deserves to stand on its own and be much more widely read and discussed than it is at present, perhaps because it is hidden within the voluminous *Inner Classic of the Yellow Emperor*. In addition, the material covered in this text is so deep, complex, and foreign to our modern way of thinking that I have come to accept over the years that no single translation, whether into modern Chinese or any Western language, could ever do it justice, much less make the content understandable to an uninitiated reader who does not have access to the original source text and the volumes of historical commentaries and discussions in classical Chinese. For this reason, I have chosen to incorporate both historical and modern commentaries by various specialists or "scholar-physicians," as well as my own ruminations. I see this text as a beautiful poetic distillation and manifestation of the traditional Chinese worldview of macrocosm-microcosm resonance, also known as "correlative thinking" or "five-phase correspondences," that forms the foundation of all aspects of traditional Chinese culture. As such, this text is relevant not just for clinical practitioners in the field of medicine, but also for scholars, historians, and thinkers interested in early Chinese science, cosmology, philosophy, religion, and even politics and economics. The present publication presents my humble contribution to making this important text and its underlying way of thinking and being and acting in the world more accessible to a modern audience. Like a finger pointing at the moon, though, I am keenly aware of the inherent limitations of this project, as of any work trying to bridge the huge gulf in time and space between our modern Western world and Hàn dynasty China. I see this book as just one more attempt, among a growing number of other renditions, to express the content of the *Great Treatise* in an accessible and at the same time historically and linguistically accurate rendition for a contemporary Western audience.[2]

[2] The most important other translations of this text in English include, but are not limited

The importance of the fifth chapter in the *Huáng Dì Nèi Jīng Sù Wèn* is underscored by the fact that the title marks it as a "Great Treatise"! Besides the seven *Sù Wèn* chapters that Wáng Bīng 王冰 added in his edition from 762 CE (chapters 66–71), only two chapters in the original *Sù Wèn* are titled *Dà Lùn* 大論 "Great Treatise": The present one and Chapter 2, the *Great Treatise on Attuning the Shén in Accordance with the Four Qì* (*Sì Qì Tiáo Shén Dà Lùn* 四氣調神大論). If I had to pick a single chapter in a single text on Chinese medicine to represent its basic paradigm, *Sù Wèn* Chapter 5 is the one that I would choose because it succinctly yet comprehensively expresses the way of thinking that has been the foundation of clinical practice in East Asia over more than two millennia. As I hope to demonstrate in the following pages, this statement is as true today as it was at the time of its compilation in the Hàn dynasty.

A word of warning though, for the uninitiated reader: It is not easy to access this text because its meaning is hidden, like the core of an onion or a set of Russian dolls, in innumerable progressive layers of insights that reveal themselves only over many years of studying and reading the text over and over. Like the slow extraction of nutrients that takes place in a goat's four stomachs, I sincerely hope that this book can encourage you to begin a sustained and sustaining practice of "rumination" on the classical medical texts that you may return to for the rest of your life. Both in my personal studies and in observing my students' efforts, I have found this ruminating practice to be most fruitful when done as a flexible combination of rigorous academic brain work with spacious aimless roaming, meditating, and even dream work. This text deserves more than just a single session of intellectual engagement. As you grow in your understanding of medicine, of early Chinese culture, and of the world and your place within it, so will your reading of the *Great Treatise* and the sustenance that you receive from it. And while you do this, you will

to, Elisabeth Rochat de la Vallée, *The Rhythm at the Heart of the World: Neijing Suwen Chapter 5* (Monkey Press, 2012); Paul U. Unschuld and Hermann Tessenow, *Huang Di Nei Jing Su Wen: An Annotated Translation of Huang Di's Inner Classic – Basic Questions* (University of California Press, 2011); Liansheng Wu and Qi Wu, *Yellow Emperor's Canon of Internal Medicine* (China Science and Technology Press, 2002); Ilza Veith, The Yellow Emperor's Classic of Internal Medicine (University of California Press, 2002); and Maoshing Ni, *The Yellow Emperor's Classic of Medicine: A New Translation of the Neijing Suwen with Commentary* (Shambhala, 1995).

learn not only about medicine but also about following the *Dào* of Heaven and Earth in a life of free-flowing ease; about harmonizing Yīn and Yáng in every micro- and macrocosm that you might encounter, and about cultivating your Heart and your Spirit in the tradition of the ancient Chinese sages.

Here is the way in which this process of expansion and deepening has played out in my own growing understanding of the meaning of this text: I began by reading *Sù Wèn* 5, like the rest of the *Yellow Emperor's Inner Classic*, in the conventional way as what we might call "microcosmic medicine," with a lower-case "m" to indicate the usage of medicine here in the main-stream meaning, as in this definition from the Merriam-Webster Collegiate dictionary:

> MEDICINE: The science and art of dealing with the maintenance of health and the prevention, alleviation, or cure of disease.[3]

Of course the *Yellow Emperor' Inner Classic* has a lot of valuable insights for just this kind of medicine, in particular in regards to the prevention of disease and "maintenance" of health. Perhaps one could even rephrase this last goal more optimistically as "optimization" of health, as the restoration of the perfect equilibrium of Yīn and Yáng and unhindered well-ordered flow of Qì in the human body. This last point alone constitutes a major contribution, in my eyes, to our global contemporary understanding of medicine and of the role of the physician, with significant potential for changing our dominant medical paradigm. This is also the way in which the *Great Treatise on the Resonant Manifestations of Yīn and Yáng* is generally read and interpreted, and applied by Chinese medicine students and practitioners both in Asia and in the West.

What I have learned over these past few months of working intensely and deeply with the meaning of the text, however, is that its core message is one of "Medicine," of medicine with a capital M. The Yellow Emperor and Qí Bó are not just talking about sticking needles into people to resolve blockages, getting enough sleep in the winter and exercise in the summer, or eliminating greasy foods and increasing the consumption of greens in the spring. As powerful as those simple messages are, this book is talking about what I now call

[3] www.merriam-webster.com/dictionary/medicine, Dec. 10, 2017.

"macrocosmic Medicine." Its teachings ARE Medicine, in the sense of the word *yào* 藥 that I am discussing below. The macrocosmic Medicine presented in the book in your hand encapsulates a vision of the role of humanity that is diametrically opposed to the paradigm of control and dominance that we see playing out all around us right now, with usually disastrous consequences: in our standard technological responses to environmental crises like global warming, exploitation of natural resources, international conflicts, punitive political responses like the "War on Drugs," incarceration rates, social hierarchical relations in the family and workplace, our relationships to our plant, animal, rock, and spirit neighbors on this plant, and also in standard biomedical solutions like cancer treatments. One only needs to look at the cardboard shacks under the highway bridges of any big city in the US to see the results of this paradigm of dominance. Can we really not do better than this?

In the place of this relatively modern ideal of humans conquering and dominating our natural environment, the Yellow Emperor and Qí Bó propose a paradigm of reciprocity, of mutual responsibility and care-taking where we humans are positioned at the center of the cosmic dyad of Heaven and Earth. Completing the macrocosmic triad, it is our role to harmonize these two and create a dynamic equilibrium of giving and taking in ecological, social, and spiritual terms. How do we get there? How do we acquire the skills necessary for macrocosmic diagnosis and treatment? Here we can turn to my favorite philosopher Zhuāngzi, whom you will encounter many more times throughout this book. In his view, it is the nature of humans to position themselves happily between Heaven and Earth, just like it is the nature of fish to swim and of birds to fly, and of old gnarly trees to provide shade for the lumber jack who is taking a nap underneath it. In sharp contrast to our current activist pursuit of visible, measurable, and quantifiable progress with instant concrete solutions, of "DOING" things and judging their effectiveness and value, the ancient Chinese sages envision a state of quietude, receptivity, humbleness, and emptiness, where simple solutions work best and where less is more and more is less. We only need to look at the history of humans on this planet, from the ancient grazing landscapes in the Swiss Alps to the steps of Mongolia and rice paddies in Southern China, to the open park-like birch forests described by the first colonists in what is now the United States of America to know that a different way of being is possible. Civilizations have come and gone, but all over the world we can find examples of humans who have lived sustainably and in harmony with our environment and our animal and plant siblings for centuries, if not millennia. Even the development of domesticated species like goats or corn or apples bear witness to the ability of humans to give and take in a mutually beneficial relationship of symbiosis with other species. We are all related to everything else through the web of Qì, after all, through breathing and eating, inside and outside our skin, living and dying, contracting and expanding. All life is Qì, and your Qì is my Qì is the Qì of the universe. So simple, and yet so easy to forget.

It is my hope that the present text can remind, encourage, and guide us to live in accordance with our original human role between Heaven and Earth by deciphering the cosmic Dào, the Way of Change as expressed through the fluctuations of Yīn and Yáng, and take us back to a simpler life in harmony with our environment. We might be well advised to heed this wisdom from the past and honor the experience of the ancient Chinese sages, who may know a thing or two that could be helpful for us, if we recognize the cyclical pattern of history and time. As we listen to them, we might learn that this path does not need to be as complicated as the invention of zero-pollution electric cars or establishing colonies on distant planets to dump our toxic waste. The simple act of feeding a hummingbird can heal our sense of estrangement from the rest of the world, our "species loneliness." Rather than running around "doing," this book is an invitation to slow down, to "un-do" and "un-know," and to contemplate another approach to life in all its dimensions. For inspiration, here is a description of the enlightened sages from *Sù Wèn* 1, the "Treatise on Heavenly Perfection in the Ancient Past" (*Shàng Gǔ Tiān Zhēn Lùn* 上古天真論)

> 夫上古聖人之教下也, 皆謂之虛邪賊風, 避之有時, 恬憺虛無, 真氣從之, 精神內守, 病安從來。
>
> 是以志閑而少欲, 心安而不懼, 形勞而不倦, 氣從以順, 各從其欲, 皆得所願。
>
> 故美其食, 任其服, 樂其俗, 高下不相慕, 其民故曰朴。

是以嗜欲不能勞其目，淫邪不能惑其心，愚智賢不肖不懼於物，故合於道。

所以能年皆度百歲，而動作不衰者，以其德全不危也。

Now in the ancient past, the ancients instructed those below them always by framing it in terms of Vacuity Evil and Bandit Wind, which must be avoided at the [necessary] times. In a state of tranquility and ease, of emptiness and absence [of desires and external stimulation], the Perfected Qì goes along with it. With the jīngshén (Essence Spirt) safeguarded inside, where could disease possibly come from?

As a result of this, their Will was at leisure and marked by few desires, their Heart was peaceful and without nervousness, their Form was taxed without being exhausted. The Qì followed along and therefore flowed in the proper direction. They each followed their desires and always obtained what they wished for.

Therefore, they took delight in their food, viewed their clothes as flattering, and took pleasure in the common. The elevated people and their inferiors did not envy each other, and the population was therefore called "in their perfect natural state."

As a result of this, their cravings and desires were not able to tax their eyes, and wanton evils were not able to confuse their Hearts. Whether they were fools or sages, paragons of virtue or prodigal children, they were not intimidated by anything. Thus they blended with the Dào.

The reason why they were all able to pass through a hundred years in age without weakening in their activity is that they kept their Virtue complete instead of endangering it.

As a whole, the *Great Treatise on the Resonant Manifestations of Yīn and Yáng* discusses the correlations and correspondences, or in my favorite translation "resonances" (*yìng* 應), between the actions and movements of Yīn and Yáng in the macrocosm of nature at large and in the human body and an infinity of other larger and smaller microcosms, from the cells to plants and animals to society and the stars in the sky. Without going into too much detail here, I would like to suggest that what English-speaking scholars of philosophy, science, and medicine have been referring to as "correlative thinking" or as the "theory of systematic correspondences" deserves a stronger and more concise term to describe this relationship of "stimulus and response/resonance" *gǎn yìng* 感應. After years of waffling, I have chosen the translation "resonance" to describe the interactions of the various microcosms with each other and with the macrocosm. I am indebted to countless esteemed Chinese medicine colleagues, teachers and students, for decades of conversations about this theme, but in particular to the three senior doctors Z'ev Rosenberg, Long Rihui, and Brenda Hood.

In addition, my reasoning has developed partly as the result of my work with this text and my efforts at explaining it to students, but also through my work with bees in my orchard; my personal experience of the effects of PTSD and of treatments with tuning forks and shamanic drumming on my nervous system and my *shén* Spirit, Qì, and *jīng* Essence; my musical training and passion as a classical violinist and twangy Mexican-style accordion player; and perhaps most importantly the lessons I learned as a biodynamic farmer, irrigating a very special piece of land in the high mountains of northern New Mexico. Most readers may be familiar with the important etymology of the Chinese character for "medicinal/remedy" *yào* 藥: It is a combination of the grass radical (signifying most likely that the first cures were primarily plant-based) on top of the character *yùe / lè* 樂 , which depicts a wooden rack with bells, drums, or jade sound stones attached to it.

Carrying the basic meanings of "music" and "joy," this character is explained in the *Yùe Jì* 樂記 (Record of Music), a chapter in the *Lǐ Jì* 禮記 (Record of Rituals) as follows:

感於物而動，故形於聲。聲相應，故生變；變成方，謂之音；比音而樂之，及干戚羽旄，謂之樂。

Sound (shēng 聲) is produced by a response to being moved by things. Sounds resonating with each other (xiāng yìng 相應) engender change. As change becomes directional (fāng 方), it produces tones. The aligning of tones and resulting music/joy, affecting shields and axes, plumes and ox-tails, this is what we call "music."

The earliest Chinese dictionary *Shuō Wén Jiě Zì* 說文解字 (Explaining Graphs and Elucidating Characters), which dates from the second century CE, explains the use of the element 樂 in the character 藥 as simply the phonetic element. Nevertheless, the choice does suggest the affinity of the early Chinese conception of medicine with the idea of resonance or vibrations, as experienced with musical instruments like bells or drums. Of course this connection makes perfect sense when we consider the all-important role of Qì in any traditional Chinese treatment, whether with medicinals, acupuncture, moxibustion, incantations, prayers, or exorcisms in a continuum of what we might for lack of a better choice call "natural" and "supernatural," or "physical" and "spiritual" modalities. Like hopefully many of my readers, I personally have had the great fortune numerous times of experiencing the calm joyful state of being in a dynamically vibrating equilibrium in perfect attunement with the environment as the result of a skillful acupuncture treatment, early-morning qigong session by the sea, or in the midst of playing chamber music. And one of the closest metaphors that comes to my mind to describe this state is the sound and feeling of universal humming in the midst of a swarm of bees. It is for this reason that I have chosen the whimsical word "humming" to translate the character *yìng* 應 in the Chinese title of the text as part of the title of the present book. For an explanation for the appearance of elephants, continue reading.

Following a commentary by Wú Kūn 吳崑 from 1594, we may often be tempted to equate Yīn and Yáng in the macrocosm in its narrowest physiological sense with Blood and Qì, respectively, in the body, especially if we approach this text narrowly as clinical medical literature without taking into consideration its early Chinese cultural context and the significance and meaning of medicine and healing within that culture. Nevertheless, I would argue that that interpretation is only one of many frames of references and will be too limiting for many passages in this chapter. As the reader will notice, the text constantly shifts between the macrocosmic view (of the Supreme Ultimate, or *tài jí* 太極) and its expression in the two-fold complementary actions of Yīn and Yáng, alternately expressed at the level of Heaven and Earth, as the unfathomable (*shén* 神) and the apparent (*míng* 明) in the phenomenal world of the Myriad Things (*wàn wù* 萬物), as the Qì and Flavor (*wèi* 味) in food and medicinal substances, or in the many correspondences of Yīn and Yáng within the human body, which, as its own macrocosm, incorporates countless more possible microcosmic systems.

The character xiàng 象, which I have chosen to render as "manifestations" throughout this book, literally means "elephant," or specifically ivory. It is an important term in early Chinese thought and requires much more time and space than I can dedicate to it in the context of this book to plumb its full meaning. For readers familiar with the *Yì Jīng* 易經 (Classic of Changes), it might be helpful to recall that *xiàng* refers to the "image" or "illustration" of the hexagrams, i.e., their visual and symbolic representation. In Chinese astrology, *tiān xiàng* 天象 refers to the celestial images or traces in the movement of the heavenly bodies that correlate with or reflect the visible phenomena on Earth. In this context, the character 象 is often paired and at the same time contrasted in a typical Yīn-Yáng duality with the term *xíng* 形, which I translate in the following pages as "Form," as the earthly manifestations of heavenly images. In this combination, *xiàng* can perhaps be seen as the formless archetypal patterns of change in the interaction of Yīn and Yáng that are associated with the ineffable nature of Heaven. Through the continuous and dynamic interaction of Yīn and Yáng, ascending and descending between Heaven and Earth, these *xiàng* take on concrete shape in their Form (*xíng*) as the Myriad Things. Moving on from the duality of Yīn and Yáng to the trinity of Heaven, Earth, and Humanity, we can now begin to contemplate the role of humans as the intermediary between these two poles in a political and cosmological sense. The opposing yet complementary forces of Yīn and Yáng need to be managed, regulated, or "put in good order" (*zhì* 治) by the ruler and sage in the socio-political realm. This involves harmonizing the country, rooting out disorder in all its manifestations, and aligning human activity with the daily, seasonal, yearly, and astrological cycles of the macrocosm. In its perhaps oldest and original sense, *zhì* 治 is the action of managing the waterways to prevent flooding in one area and drought in the other, as the mythical culture hero Yǔ 禹, tamer of floods and founder of China's first Xià dynasty, is said to have done. It is no coincidence, however, that the same character that is used to describe this activity of the ruler in ruling or "putting in good order" the country (*zhì guó* 治國) is also used in the compound *zhì bìng* 治病, "to treat disease," which is the activity of the medical practitioner. The overlap and complementarity between the two microcosms of the body politic and the human body are well-known to any student of Chinese medicine or culture. As in the case of ruling the country, the physician is also in charge of "managing the waterways," in this case by promoting free flow (of Qì and Blood), avoiding pathological blockages, and ensuring the healthy movement of vital substances in and out and up and down and through the entirety of the human body. In my mind, the *Great Discourse on the Resonant Manifestations of Yīn and Yáng* is the perfect expression of this basic identity between the activities of the sage-ruler and the sage-physician, riding the Dào by following the flow in the right direction (*shùn* 順) in the ever-moving currents of Yīn-Yáng change. Enjoy, be inspired, and learn!

I have not chosen this project lightly and have utmost respect and love for this text in its original language. Therefore, I have resisted a formal translation project for years and have then spent the past few years exploring different formats and approaches on how to create a useful contribution to the growing secondary literature on the *Great Treatise* and the *Yellow Emperor's Inner Classic* as a whole. This manuscript has undergone many, many revisions and transformations, and will always be far from perfect. But at some point, any writer or creative person must find a productive balance between their urge for perfection (and fear of imperfection and resulting criticism) and the need to share what they are able to create with a broader public audience who may benefit from this work. It is my hope that I have struck that balance with this book in its current format, and that my baby, after a long hard labor, is now ready to see the light of day and say hello to the rest of the world.

ORGANIZATION OF THIS BOOK

The layout of this book has undergone many alterations in an effort to balance readability and accessibility with the need to stay true to the original source text. The current form of the translation, commentaries, and discussion below has been chosen intentionally and carefully to guide readers back to the original source whenever possible, and to clearly differentiate between the original text and various interpretations. The admittedly ambitious underlying intention has been to create a translation that is meaningful both to those readers who have no background at all in classical Chinese and to those who might know some modern or minimal classical Chinese. In the hope of inspiring more practitioners of Chinese medicine to take up the study of the classical language, I have made every attempt to indicate grammatical structures, explain any deviations from the most literal reading in my English translations, and discuss alternative readings and my reasons for privileging one over another when appropriate. To assist the reader in pairing the Chinese source with my literal translation, I have broken the Chinese up into sections and lines, and added punctuation. In this practice, I have mostly followed my Chinese predecessors, alerting the reader on alternative readings as necessary. In addition, I have found it increasingly necessary, over years of working with this text and communicating my understanding of it to students with sometimes little background in classical Chinese culture, to elaborate on important medical concepts, cultural values, philosophical terms, and even grammatical and linguistic explorations in sometimes lengthy detours. My intention is simply to make this important text as accessible as possible to readers who may not be able to appreciate its deeper layers of meaning without this sort of guidance and explanation. Unable to hold each of you hostage in my living room for a month, maybe this book will at least whet your appetite for the Chinese classics and stimulate you to explore other texts or aspects of this tradition in the future.

FREQUENTLY CITED SOURCES AND COMMENTARIES

The following commentaries and interpretations, in English and in Chinese, are cited throughout the book and provided a starting point for my understanding of this text. Given the great age of the *Huáng Dì Nèi Jīng* and the well-known problems with any of the received versions of the text, my translation does rely on historical interpretations. To do otherwise would be arrogance and folly. My decades of working with this text have taught me to respect the accumulated wisdom of two thousand years of Chinese scholarship and clinical expertise, which in my case was complemented perfectly by the contemporary teachings of Dr. Rihui Long at the National University of Natural Medicine in Portland, Oregon, based on his own training in Nèijīng Studies in China and a rich lifetime of clinical experience. The sources below are, after the first occurrence, referred to merely by the author's name. Other sources are cited in full as they occur throughout the book.

- GĀO SHÌZŌNG 高士宗, *Huáng Dì Sù Wèn Zhí Jiě* 《黄帝素問直解》 (Straightforward Explanations of the *Huáng Dì Sù Wèn*).

- ELISABETH ROCHAT DE LA VALLÉE, *The Rhythm at the Heart of the World: Neijing Suwen Chapter 5* (Monkey Press, 2012).

- PAUL U. UNSCHULD AND HERMANN TESSENOW, *Huang Di Nei Jing Su Wen: An Annotated Translation of Huang Di's Inner Classic – Basic Questions* (University of California Press, 2011.

- WÚ KŪN 吳崑, *Sù Wèn Wú Zhù* 《素問吳注》 (Commentary by Wú Kūn on the *Plain Questions*).

- ZHĀNG JIÈBĪN 張介賓, *Lèi Jīng* 《類經》 (Categorized Classic).

- ZHĀNG ZHÌCŌNG 張志聰, *Huáng Dì Nèi Jīng Sù Wèn Jí Zhù*《黄帝內經素問集注》(Collected Commentaries on the *Yellow Emperor's Inner Classic, Plain Questions).*

Quotations that are identified as "Commentaries" by historical authors in the following pages are culled from medical writings that were composed as commentaries on specific lines of the *Great Treatise*. The critical reader may rest assured that I have taken care to never quote them out of context but always place them next to the line that they comment on. In addition, I have followed the practice of Chinese commentators and often complemented my discussion with quotations from other sources, medical, philosophical, or otherwise. Please note that these writings might bear no direct relation to the *Nèi Jīng* in their original context and were randomly selected by me to shed light on certain terms or concepts. These I have identified below as "Quotations." At times, my choice of supplementary material has been influenced by references to these texts in earlier *Nèi Jīng* commentaries but more often they are simply passages from the classics that I have used in my classes to illustrate a certain concept or point. My intention with this structure is twofold: first, I have attempted to replicate the traditional Chinese way of studying, reading, and writing about this text, which has always been done by relying on the explanations of previous commentators.[4] Second, this format expresses my own style of lecturing in person that I have developed over years of teaching this material, especially in the framework of the Classical Texts series at the College of Classical Chinese Medicine at the National University of Natural Medicine in Portland, Oregon. It is thus the closest equivalent to a seminar-style discussion that I have been able to create.

HOW TO USE THIS BOOK

The following conventions have been adopted for the sake of clarity and convenience:

- *Tǔ* 土 and *dì* 地 are both translated as "earth" but *tǔ* 土 "earth" is not capitalized, while *dì* 地 "Earth," as a counterpart to *tiān* 天 "Heaven," is. If I were writing this book in a vacuum, I would have chosen "soil" as a translation of *tǔ* 土 to avoid this potential for confusion. But alas, this book is written for readers with some background knowledge in Chinese medicine who will most likely be well-steeped in the vocabulary of what is still most commonly known as the "Five Elements": Wood – Fire – Earth – Metal – Water. I wanted to make sure that such readers recognize *tǔ* as one of these "Five Elements" (or in my rendering "dynamic agents").

[4] For an excellent example of this style of reading the *Nèi Jīng*, see Elisabeth Hsu, *The Transmission of Chinese Medicine*, Chapter Four on "Interpreting a classical Chinese medical text," 105-127.

- Technical terms are capitalized to alert the reader that their usage here differs from the standard usage in the English language.

- Chinese terms are transcribed in Pīnyīn, intoned, and in italics, unless they are either commonly known terms like Qì, Yīn, and Yáng, which I treat as English words, or proper names of decoctions, persons, places, etc. Book titles are capitalized and italicized.

- For ease of reading and aesthetics, I have minimized the use of footnotes, in comparison to more academic publications, and refer the reader to the list of references in the Appendix for full bibliographical information on all sources used in this book.

To slow all of us down and encourage us to step back from a purely intellectual engagement with the text, we have added some illustrations. As mentioned above, this text is as inadequate in conveying the full message of the ancients as is the finger pointing at the moon or the description of an apple to somebody who has never touched or tasted one. We very much hope that you will read this book slowly and in chunks, interspersed with frequent walks, naps, dreams, art sessions, contemplation of sunsets and sunrises, smelling of a rose, or at least many steaming cups of Pu'er tea in happy company, to follow the example of the ancient Chinese sages. The translation and transmission of the ancient Chinese teachings on medicine and the cosmos is truly a work in progress, one that has been carried on for countless generations by countless individuals and groups. May this book serve as a small piece in that grand puzzle...

Acknowledgments

My understanding of the *Great Treatise* has benefited immensely from the penetrating wisdom, clinical explanations, good humor, philosophical depth, comprehensive scholarship, and profound humanity of Dr. Long Rihui, greatly beloved teacher emeritus at the National University of Natural Medicine. The spirit of his teachings, based on a lifetime of clinical practice and dedication to transmitting his knowledge, shines throughout this book. I had the great honor of learning from and teaching with him for two years in small doctoral seminars on the *Huáng Dì Nèi Jīng*, taught as part of the Classical Texts curriculum at the College of Classical Chinese Medicine at the National University of Natural Medicine.

My deep gratitude also to the many brilliant, dedicated, enthusiastic, critical, and compassionate students who have joined me on my journey of working with this text. Your questions, insights, struggles, and successes have inspired me to attempt to share what we learned together in class with a broader audience through this book. May we always continue to inspire each other in our shared journey of lifelong learning with passion, dedication, heart, and laughter.

In addition, I want to thank my many wonderful clinical colleagues in the field of Chinese medicine, but Drs. Z'ev Rosenberg and Brenda Hood in particular, for their assistance in wrapping my head around the meaning of "resonance" in Chinese medicine over many years of shared conversations about harmony, music, healing, and the universe. I count myself so fortunate to be working in a profession overflowing with genuinely lovely and loving human beings who are so generous in sharing what they know with this strange academic nerd in their midst. Of course all the mistakes in this book are my own.

During my first year in college in Germany, when I first reluctantly accepted the fact that I dearly love dead languages and philosophy in spite of my vivacious personality, I could never have imagined that I would get to actually bring this material to life with the help of passionate readers and audiences who care this much about my obscure research and strange writings. It is a rare gift for an academic, especially one working in a dead language, to have engaged readers like you, who send me sweet notes of appreciation and leave me gifts of Elsatian butter and lavender oil after seminars. I never take you for granted, and it is your interest that has given me the courage and strength to take on and carry through this project. And it was your feedback on how the information in the classics is making a difference in your clinical practice and personal and professional lives that convinced me of the need for this book in the first place.

Last but definitely not least, I want to thank my fantastic publishing team at Happy Goat Productions, without whom I would have never dreamed of taking on this project. This includes three outstanding clinical consultants and scholar-physicians of the highest caliber: Brenda Hood who has generously answered innumerable clinical questions and also provided steadfast encouragement, honest constructive criticism and challenging questions, and unconditional friendship of the highest kind, and Leo Lok and Z'ev Rosenberg who have read and commented on this manuscript in its various incarnations and supported me at times when I was ready to give up. Z'ev Rosenberg in particular has added immensely to this project with his foreword and the succinct clinical commentaries found throughout the book. Sue Minger for being the essential cheer-leading part of the team on Whidbey Island; Keith Schreiber (www.jkschreiber.com), Remee Gemo (www.remee.gallery), and Sunjae Lee (www.fermatawellness.com) for so generously sharing their art work and thereby adding a very special touch to this book:

Keith provided the stunning photography for the background images of the Section pages, Remee the gorgeous image for the book cover, and Sunjae a few paintings throughout the book. Lillian Pearl Bridges! Without your love, wisdom, example, and compassionate encouragement I would never have had the strength and courage to wholeheartedly dedicate myself to my "Golden Path" and make room for this work in my life. You have also kept me well fed and happy. Lastly, we are so fortunate to have Barbara Tada on the team, our wonderful graphic designer whose clear and clean sense of aesthetic is responsible for the visual beauty of this book. It takes a very special combination of skills to have mastered the complex layout for this book with so many layers of Chinese and English text and commentary, notes and discussion, which is something I know nothing about. I am so grateful for your professional dedication and perfectionism, elegant sense of aesthetic, and willingness to manifest my vision in a concrete book.

Part One

Macrocosmic & Microcosmic Interactions of Yīn & Yáng

Section One

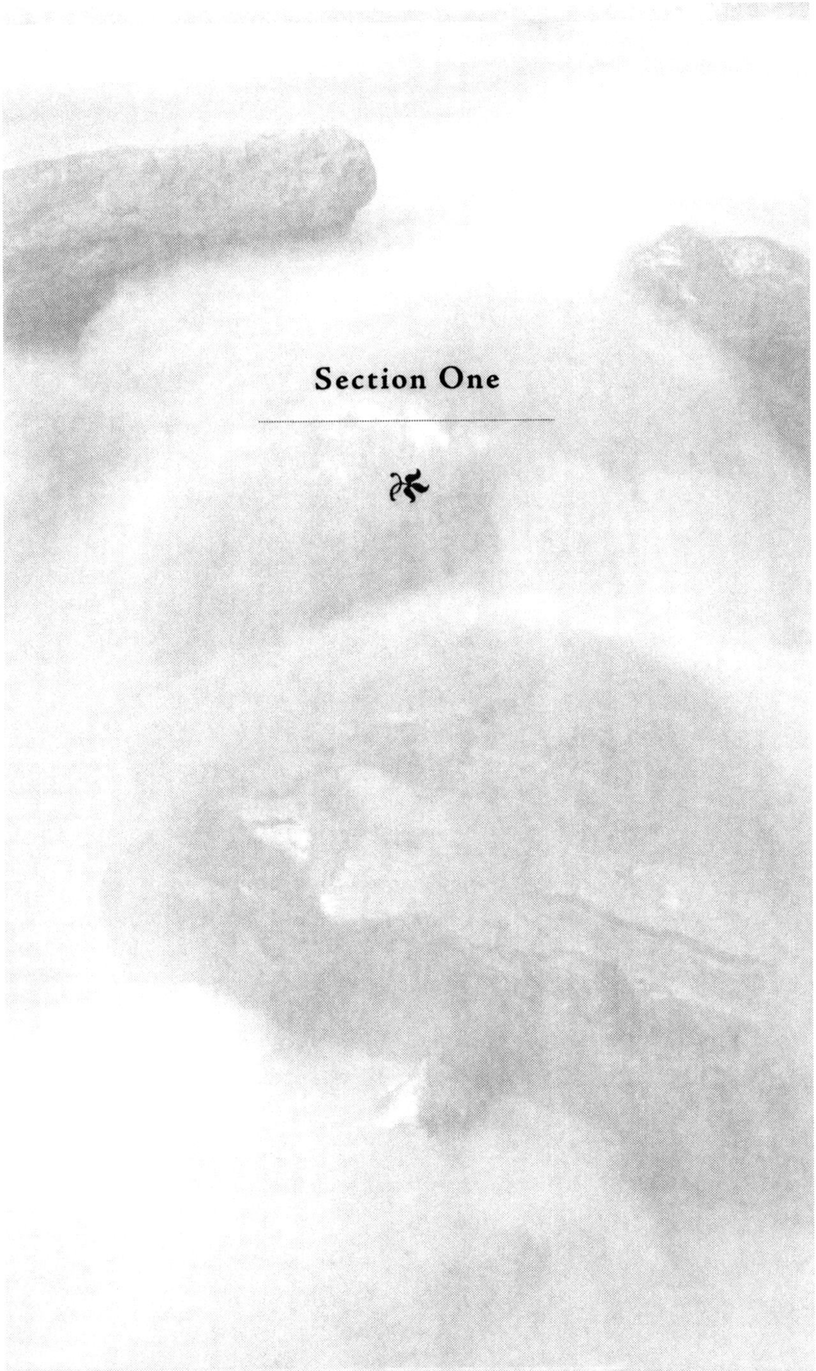

黃帝曰：陰陽者，天地之道也，萬物之綱紀，變化之父母，生殺之本始，神明之府也。

Huáng dì yuē: Yīn yáng zhě,
tiān dì zhī dào yě, wàn wù zhī gang jì,
biàn huà zhī fù mǔ, shēng shā zhī
běn shǐ, shén míng zhī fǔ yě.

The Yellow Emperor said:
"Yīn and Yáng! They are the Dào of Heaven and Earth! They are the guide ropes and connecting threads of the Myriad Things, the father and mother of Alterations and Transformations, the foundation and beginning of giving birth and taking life, and the Palace of the *shén míng*.

Commentary by Zhāng Jièbīn 張介賓[1]

道者，陰陽之理也。陰陽者，一分為二也。太極動而生陽，靜而生陰，天生於動，地生於靜，故陰陽為天地之道。

The Dào! It is the guiding principle of Yīn and Yáng. Yīn and Yáng are the One divided into Two. In activity, the Supreme Ultimate (tàijí) engenders Yáng; in stillness, it engenders Yīn. Heaven is engendered through activity; Earth is engendered through stillness. Hence Yīn and Yáng are the Dào of Heaven and Earth.

IT WOULD BE EASY FOR ME TO FILL AN ENTIRE BOOK WITH AN exploration of this line alone, and still I would fail to express its meaning adequately. This opening statement is the perfect example of how I hope to engage the reader with this book: My ruminations are intended as just a start, an entryway into *Nèi Jīng* studies that will entice all of us to spend many more years immersed in the study of the literary language, cosmology, philosophy, and medicine that the ancient texts express so beautifully. Words can only take us so far on this path. Eventually, each of us reaches the limit of our rational understanding and is forced to switch to non-rational ways of making sense of the world, whether through art, meditation, contemplation of nature, medical experience, or your own way that I may not be able to relate to but that will move you along this path.

Throughout this entire book, it is essential to keep in mind the grand topic and underlying theme, as expressed in this first line: the discussion of Yīn and Yáng as the "Dào of Heaven and Earth," to be grasped in its myriad manifestations from the macrocosm down to the tiniest microcosms through the "resonances" or "echoes" (*yìng* 應) that can be perceived everywhere that we care to focus our senses on. These

[1] Zhāng Jièbīn 張介賓, *Lèi Jīng* 《類經》 (Categorized Classic, 1624).

"resonances" are like the responding vibrations that the powerful beat on a large drum causes in a small drum, which is actually one of the alternate definitions of the character *yìng* in the chapter title that I have rendered as "resonance" but that is more commonly translated as "correspondence." After years of teaching Chinese medicine students the basics about Yīn and Yáng and what is usually called "correlative thinking" or "Five-Element correspondences" in English, I have learned to emphasize the key difference between mere "correlation" or "association" and actual "resonance." In Chinese medicine, the Heart is not just "associated with" or "related to" Fire and summer, and the Kidney to Water and winter, but literally and very physically affected by it. As such, the internal organs in the human body and its associated emotions, physical constituents, sensory organs etc., change in direct and observable response to seasonal cycles, diet, astronomical events, and other micro- or macrocosmic fluctuations or happenings. All of these ceaseless changes are summarized in the *Nèi Jīng* as the "Dào of Heaven and Earth." And the ability of the sage and visionary to interpret past changes, read the present, and thereby predict future changes is the key to a successful life as a human in between Heaven and Earth, whether as the ruler of a country, an immortal in the mountains, or a physician and master of "nurturing life" (*yǎng shēng* 養生).

Returning to the first line of the "Great Discourse on the Resonant Manifestations of Yīn and Yáng," a bit of additional explanation on a few terms and characters can help us gain a deeper level of understanding than a cursory reading of the simple literal translation would allow: The phrase gāng *jì* 綱紀 consists of two technical terms that refer to the two types of rope that make up a fishing net, one the stronger guide rope on the top to encircle and enclose the net and the other the smaller strands that form the actual net. In its use in the present context, the expression is generally interpreted as a compound along the lines of "fundamental principles" or "laws and principles."[2] Looked at in more detail as two separate terms, however, we can read

[2] Unschuld and Tessenow, *Huang Di Nei Jing Su Wen: An Annotated Translation of Huang Di's Inner Classic – Basic Questions*, 95, and Rochat de la Vallée, *The Rhythm at the Heart of the World: Neijing Suwen Chapter 5*, 13.

the two characters more specifically as both the general principles or guidelines for understanding the universe (the "guide rope" that holds the net together at the top and allows the fisher to grasp the entirety of the catch) as well as the detailed standards to measure specific manifestations thereof (the "connecting threads" that make up the bulk and structure of the actual net and in conceptual terms provide the fine details, perhaps less glamorous but just as essential as the grand principles). As so often in literary Chinese, this pair of terms provides a sort of Yīn and Yáng balance between the grand and the small, the tangible and the intangible, the moving and the constant aspects of reality. To fully grasp the changes affecting the "Myriad Things," in other words the totality of our perceptible environment between Heaven and Earth, we need to pay attention not only to the grand principles that enclose the net, as it were, but also to the small details that allow the fishing net to hold anything.

Commentary by Gāo Shìzōng 高士宗[3]

萬物之多，變化出焉。物極，謂之變；物生，謂之化；變者，化之漸；化者，變之成。變化之道，本於陰陽，故陰陽者，變化之父母。

The multiplicity of the Myriad Things! All Alterations and Transformations emanate from it. The extreme state of things is what we call "alterations"; the creation of things is what we call "transformation." Alteration is the gradual aspect of Transformation; Transformation is the maturation of Alteration. It is because the Dào of all Alterations and Transformations is based in Yīn and Yáng that Yīn and Yáng are the father and mother of Alterations and Transformations.

[3] Gāo Shìzōng 高士宗, *Huáng Dì Sù Wèn Zhí Jiě* 《黃帝素問直解》 (Straightforward Explanations of the Huáng Dì Sù Wèn, Qing period).

In the next phrase, "the father and mother of Alterations and Transformations," the phrase *biàn huà* 變化, which simply means "change" in modern Chinese, is actually a reference to two specific types of change: *Huà* 化 describes sudden, irreversible, substantive, and often generative change, in the literal sense of "meta-morphosis," such as from the pupa to the butterfly, or from non-being to being. *Biàn* 變, on the other hand, refers to gradual, slow alterations, such as between Yīn and Yáng, day and night, water and ice, or seasonal changes. As the commentary *Nèi Jīng Zhī Yào* 《內經知要》 (Synopsis of the *Inner Classic*) differentiates: "Gradual [change] of things is called *biàn*, the extreme poles of things are called *huà*." According to the *Yùe Lìng* 《月令》 (Monthly Commands), a chapter of the *Lǐ Jì* 《禮記》 (Record of Rituals) from the Hàn period, "when there is an old form that very gradually changes, we call it *biàn*. When there is sudden change, even though there is an old form [to begin with], we call it *huà*. ...Sprouting [plants] in the spring and [leaves] dropping in the winter are called *biàn*, as is the change from childhood to adulthood and from adulthood to old age. From existence to non-existence or from non-existence to existence, this is *huà*."

Another option for rendering these two types of change into English may be as "permutations" and "transmutations." In this context, it is ironic that *biàn* is often translated as "to transform" in English, when it is really *huà*-type change that "transcends the form," often by bringing into being, as opposed to just altering it. The easiest way to distinguish between these two types of change is perhaps by looking at the context of their usage. The most commonly cited examples of *huà*-type change are found in the *Zhuāngzi* 莊子: the metamorphosis from the giant fish Kūn to the bird Péng, or from the dreaming *Zhuāngzi* himself into a butterfly.

Quotations from Zhuāngzi 莊子[4]

北冥有魚、其名爲鯤。鯤之大、不知其幾千里也。化而爲鳥、其名爲鵬。
鵬之背、不知其幾千里也。怒而飛、其翼若垂天之雲。
是鳥也、海運 則將徙於南冥。南冥者、天池也。

In the Northern Darkness, there exists a fish with the name Kūn. Kūn's size is I don't know how many thousands of miles. It transforms (huà!) into a bird with the name Péng. Péng's back is I don't know how many thousands of miles. Arousing itself and taking off in flight, its wings are like the clouds hanging from the sky. When the oceans churn, this bird migrates to the Southern Darkness. The Southern Darkness is the Pond of Heaven.

昔者莊周夢爲胡蝶，栩栩然胡蝶也，自喻適志與。不知周也。
俄然覺 則蘧蘧然周也。不知周之夢爲胡蝶與胡蝶之夢
爲周與。周與胡蝶則必有分矣。此之謂物化。

In the past, Zhuāng Zhōu dreamed that he was a butterfly, a happily fluttering butterfly who considered itself to be utterly satisfied, not knowing anything about Zhōu. Suddenly, it woke up and was pleasantly surprised to be Zhōu. Who knows whether it was Zhōu dreaming of being a butterfly or the butterfly dreaming of being Zhōu! Zhōu and the butterfly, now there must be a distinction between them! This is what is called the "transformation of things."

[4] These quotations come from Chapter 1, *Xiāo Yáo Yóu* 逍遙遊 (Free and Easy Wandering) and Chapter 2, *Qí Wù Lùn* 齊物論 (Discourse on Evening Things Out), respectively.

In contrast, *biàn* is a slow gradual change, as in weather cycles, seasonal changes, or the gradual aging of the human body. In Chinese dictionaries, the difference is explained as *biàn* being a change where the two states can be present simultaneously, like the alterations or variations between Yīn and Yáng or between day and night or winter and summer. In contrast, *huà* is a complete and irreversible substantive change from one thing into something else, like the caterpillar into the butterfly, where the two states cannot be present simultaneously, or even a coming into being. In the context of cosmology, *huà* change is the origin of creation, while *biàn* are the innumerable and never-ending cyclical alterations that are the defining characteristic of the material realm in the cycles of the Five Phases and Yīn and Yáng. Reflecting the importance of change in early Chinese culture, the medical anthropologist Elisabeth Hsu has written an entire article on these two characters: "Change in Chinese Medicine: Bian and Hua. An Anthropologist's Approach."

"In 2010, a lexicon of sea ice terminology in Nunavik, *Siku: Knowing Our Ice*, included no fewer than 93 different words. No matter the type of term it uses to refer to a particular type of snow or ice, Inuktitut has a far superior ability to distinguish between them than most languages."[5]

Note that in the following pages, *huà* often implies the meaning of "to produce through change," or even "to create." In the phrase *yáng huà qì* 陽化氣 "Yáng creates Qì" (see page 50), for example, the verb *huà* really does mean a coming into being, the production of something that did not exist previously, and I have translated it accordingly. To conclude this discussion and avoid frustration, let us just remember that different languages have different levels of specificity for terms that matter more in one culture than another.

[5] Katie D'Angelo, *30 Inuktitut Words for Snow and Ice*, Historica Canada Blog: www.historicacanada.ca/blog/30-inuktitut-words-for-snow-and-ice, Oct. 2, 2017.

So perhaps the most important message to take away is not the precise meaning of the phrase *biàn huà* here but the fact that early Chinese culture placed such an emphasis on understanding change as the Essence of the universe that they needed to distinguish between different types of change with far more accuracy than we are capable of in any Western language, or even in modern Chinese.

Another phrase that is in need of an explanation is the compound *shén míng* 神明. I have actually left this term untranslated here because it is too complex of a concept to convey in a single combination of English words. And given its importance in early medical literature, it deserves some attention. In other contexts, I tend to follow the standard practice and translate *shén* 神 as "spirit" or "spirits," and *míng* 明 as "bright" or "to brighten," or "brightness." In medical and philosophical texts, *shén míng* often comes close in meaning to the perhaps most literal English translation "spirit radiance," and may even express an actual physical halo-like light, or at least the "illuminated" state, of certain individuals who have attained a high level of self-cultivation. But what precisely does this mean?

Looking at the etymology of the characters, *shén* 神 is a combination of the radical 示 ("altar" or any place where sacrifices are offered to the ancestors) and the phonetic 申 (two hands stretched upward). The whole character thus has the connotation of stretching and reaching upward, presumably to Heaven, in an effort to establish sacred connection, as is done in sacrifices, which result in the bestowal of blessings when performed correctly. The term is so important and yet so difficult to render in English that most contemporary Chinese medicine practitioners simply call it "the *Shén*" in professional publications and conversations. "Spirit" or "spirits" often works quite well, except that we are forced in English to either make it a singular or plural term when the Chinese encompasses both of these meanings at the same time: Our consciousness, the vitality that is reflected in our eyes when we are alive and "full of spirit," which we might be tempted to write with a capital "S," but at the same time also the many spirits that inhabit our body and the world around us and connect us to Heaven. Whether we read it as singular or plural, it is significant that it is housed in the Heart and that, in the meaning of "spirits," it is often paired in a Yīn-Yáng combination with the term *guǐ* 鬼, which is usually translated as "ghosts." While *shén* "spirit/s" is associated with Yáng and with Heaven, *guǐ* "ghost/s" is associated with Yīn and with Earth. Used as an adjective, the character carries the meaning of "spiritual," "divine," or "sacred," but can also be used to describe something that transcends ordinary human experience or capabilities.

* * *

Quotation from Zhuāngzi 莊子[6]

聖人休，休焉則平易矣，平易則恬惔矣。平易恬惔，
則憂患不能入，邪氣不能襲，故其德全而神不虧。

The sage rests. Resting then results in balance and ease. Balance and ease then result in tranquil indifference. Balance, ease, and tranquil indifference mean that worries and trouble are unable to enter and that evil qi is unable to carry out a sneak attack. For this reason, the sage's virtue/power is complete and the Shén is/are not lost.

* * *

Míng 明, THE SECOND CHARACTER IN THE COMPOUND *SHÉN MÍNG* 神明, is simply a combination of 日 (sun) and 月 (moon) and hence indicates the notion of light or brightness, as symbolized by the two brightest bodies in the sky. On the basis of this literal meaning, it can be used as a verb in the causative sense meaning "to make something bright," i.e., to explain or shed light on something," or in the putative sense as "to consider something bright." In other words, *míng* as a verb can refer to emitting light, to light shining out from an object and onto other things, or to receiving light, to light being shined onto an object. Like the English "bright" but often with a more powerful positive connotation, it is used in the metaphorical sense to refer to something that is clearly apparent and shining forth for all to see, like

[6] *Zhuāngzi* 《莊子》 Chapter 15, *Kè Yì* 刻意 (Carved Intention).

the ruler's wisdom or virtue. As the famous text *Dà Xué* 《大學》 (Great Learning) begins, "The Dào of Great Learning lies in making bright virtue shine forth" (大學之道在明明德). Reflecting the importance of perception, of seeing and understanding the true nature of things in the ever-changing flow of the Dào, *míng* is thus a key term used frequently to describe the sage, the ruler, and the healer.

To grasp the full meaning of *míng* in the compound *shén míng*, we might have to suspend our need in the English language to decide between "emitting light" and "receiving light," and therefore leave the term untranslated. The reader is invited to attempt to hold both meanings at the same time, that of the spirit/s shining brightly from within and that of the spirit/s being illuminated from without and reflecting the light of the sun and moon through the connection with Heaven. Ultimately, these need to be comprehended as the same thing.

In pharmaceutical literature, the phrase *shén míng* describes the effect of certain medicinals, specifically ones that are taken long-term in an alchemical context. In the *Shén Nóng Běncǎo Jīng* 神農本草經 (Divine Farmer's Classic of Materia Medica), for example, we commonly encounter the phrase *tōng shén míng* 通神明, which I eventually ended up rendering quite awkwardly as "facilitating the break-through of spirit illumination" in my published translation of this text.[7] As a brave effort to translate *shén míng* for non-medical readers of early Chinese literature, Paul Kroll's *Student's Dictionary of Classical and Medieval Chinese* offers "divinely luminous Essences" as a translation for this compound and explains it as "all spiritual entities amidst Heaven and Earth, from spirits to natural objects to body-gods to transcendent beings of practical immortality."[8] To return to translations of the passage discussed in the present book, Paul U. Unschuld and Hermann Tessenow's "spirit brilliance" nicely complements Elisabeth Rochat de la Vallée's "radiance of the spirits."[9]

[7] See Wilms, *The Divine Farmer's Classic of Materia Medica*, 10-12.

[8] Kroll, *A Student's Dictionary of Classical and Medieval Chinese*, 407.

[9] Unschuld and Tessenow, 95, and Rochat de la Vallée, 13.

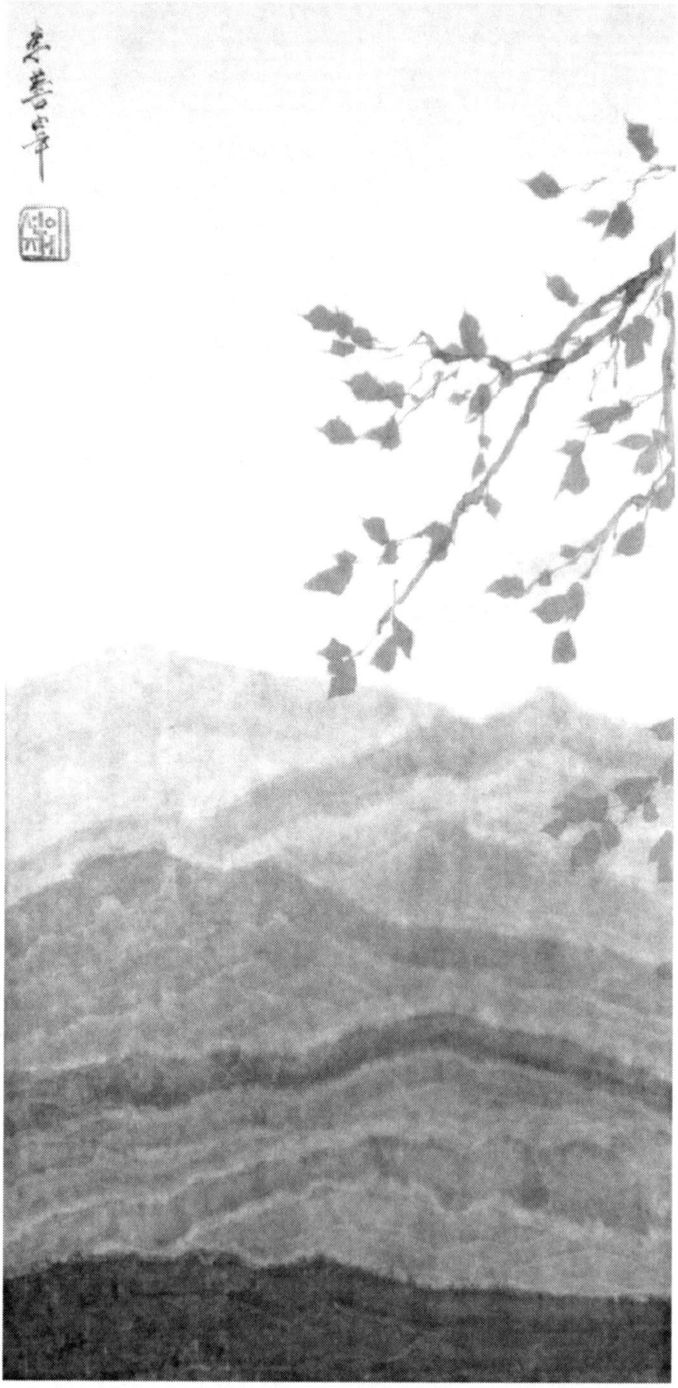

Now, however, I need to complicate things further and offer yet another possible interpretation of the compound *shén míng*, one that is cited by most Chinese commentators but ignored in all English translations that I am aware of: This definition comes from the *Xì Cí Zhùan* 《繫辭傳》 (Commentary on the Appended Phrases), a commentary on the *Yì Jīng* 《易經》 (Book of Changes): "What is immeasurable/unfathomable in Yīn and Yáng is called *Shén*; what is clearly apparent on the outside in affairs and things is called *míng*" (陰陽不測謂之神；事物照章謂之明). As such, the compound *shén míng*, at least in the minds of traditional Chinese readers of the *Nèi Jīng*, also refers to both the ineffable dimensions of Yīn and Yáng and the visible manifestations of their interplay in all perceptible things and actions.

All that being said, what do we now take away as the meaning of this statement that Yīn and Yáng are the "palace of the *shén míng*"? If you have been reading this far in the hope of getting an answer, I must disappoint you, dear reader. It is far from my intention to tell anybody else what this expression means. I invite you to contemplate the various dimensions of the terms that I have introduced above and then, through many more decades of studying texts and experiencing life, develop your own ever-deepening understanding of Yīn and Yáng as the "palace of the *shén míng*."

治病必求於本。

Zhì bìng bì qiú yú běn.

To treat disease, you must seek it in the basics.

* * *

Commentary by Zhāng Jièbīn 張介賓

本，致病之原也。人之疾病，或在表，或在裡，或為寒，或為熱，或感於五運六氣，或傷於臟腑經絡，皆不外陰陽二氣，必有所本。故或本於陰，或本於陽，病變雖多，其本則一。知病所從生，知亂所由起，而直取之，是為得一之道。譬之伐木而引其柢，則千枝萬葉，莫得弗從矣。

"Basics" means the source that caused the disease. Human diseases, whether located in the exterior or in the interior, whether consisting of Cold or of Heat, whether contracted from the 'five movements and six Qì' or through injury to the Zàng and Fǔ Organs or channels and network vessels, never fall outside these two Qì of Yīn and Yáng and hence must be based in either of them. As such they can be based in Yīn or they can be based in Yáng, but regardless of how numerous the pathological alterations are, the basis is always this single [cause]. Knowing where disease sprouted from, and knowing where disorder arose from, and then directly seizing that, this is the Dào of "Obtaining the One." By analogy, if you fell a tree and pull out its taproot, none of the thousands of branches and tens of thousands of leaves are able to survive independently.

* * *

THIS FAMOUS LINE, OFTEN CITED OUT OF CONTEXT AS ONE OF THE great truisms of Chinese medicine, is usually translated along the lines of "To treat disease, seek the root." In comparison with my version above, that rendition serves as a concise and far more elegant way of summarizing Chinese medicine, especially in contrast to biomedicine, which is often said to merely address the symptoms. Given the continued centrality of this short and seemingly simple statement in Chinese medicine both in East Asia and the West, I have intentionally chosen a different version, to alert the reader to two fine points. In spite of the title of this book, the following discussion on "trunks" has nothing to do with elephant anatomy, or with men's swimwear for that matter.

Grammatically, the presence of the preposition *yú* 於 (in, on, at, by...) is significant and must not be ignored. Like the English "seek," the Chinese verb *qiú* 求 has a direct object, which in the present line is left out, as is often the case in literary Chinese when a word is considered obvious and therefore unnecessary to the author and readers. In English, grammar rules force us to complete such gaps, which I have done by adding "it." Because of the preposition *yú* 於, the noun *běn* 本, here translated as "basics," cannot function as the direct object of "to seek" but must describe a location or direction, to specify where the search for the disease should take place. I will return to the possible significance of the difference between seeking the disease in the basics versus seeking the basics and to the possible meanings of "basics" here below.

Moreover, the noun *běn* 本 can certainly carry the metaphorical meaning of "root" and tends to be translated as such in English translations of medical literature. More strictly speaking, however, and in contrast with the more specific term *gēn* 根, which does literally refer to the roots of a tree, *běn* also refers to the trunk of the tree, or perhaps when we consider the pictograph directly, the totality of the tree at its core that stretches from the very top through the branches all the way through the surface down to the roots. This is nicely reflected in the compound *biāo běn* 標本, which is usually translated in medical literature as the "root and tips" or "cause and symptoms" of a disease. Nigel Wiseman paraphrases "root and tip" as "primary and secondary aspects of disease," and explains: "The word 'root' is used in opposition to 'tip', the two terms being of varying significance according to context. Root refers to *1* the essential nature of the disease, when tip is the signs; *2* the cause of disease, when the tip is clinically observable changes in the body; *3* right qì, when the tip is the evil; or *4* the primary condition, when the tip is the resulting secondary condition."[10] Nevertheless, in this compound we are not literally looking at the top of the tree and the root in a top-down model, but rather at the tips of the branches, the most outward and visible manifestations, and the tree's trunk in the sense of its durable core in the middle.

[10] Wiseman and Feng, *A Practical Dictionary of Chinese Medicine,* 508.

Now, in a more metaphorical sense in many contexts, this concept of "trunk" is used to refer to the "foundation" of things, which is most certainly a common meaning of the character *běn* already in literary Chinese. In most such texts, *běn* is thus quite accurately translated with the more elegant English term "root." It may strike the cursory reader as splitting hairs, but in my mind, perhaps based on many years of caring for an orchard full of old trees, there is in fact a distinction to be made between looking for disease in the trunk and looking for it in the root, or even looking for the root itself. To cite just one obvious application, one can saw off a large branch or root, perhaps to isolate some rot there, without killing the tree. But a treatment for the trunk is of quite a different nature. To follow the lead of the Yellow Emperor and play out this agricultural metaphor for dealing with disorder in the body, treating disease in the *biāo*, i.e., the very ends of a tree's branches, might mean pruning those diseased parts or applying pesticides or fertilizer to the foliage. Alternately, it could also mean to allow nature to take its course and wait for the leaves to fall and winter storms to blow off the weakened twigs, thereby getting rid of the affliction. In many cases, these approaches are perfectly appropriate responses to a superficial and passing problem. Treating a problem with a tree's health through the roots, on the other hand, might mean to improve the soil that surrounds the tree, irrigating and feeding the tree through the roots, and adding mycorrhizae and fungi to enrich the tree's ability to absorb nutrients from the soil. Treating the roots alone would be a bit more limiting perhaps but certainly related, since the roots feed the trunk and thereby the entirety of the tree. The distinction between "root" and "trunk" may thus offer precious insights as we contemplate the deeper meaning of the pair *biāo* and *běn* 標本, found in the common treatment principle "simultaneous treatment of *biāo* and *běn*" (*biāo běn jiān zhì* 標本兼治) and in the line above, about managing disease by "seeking it in the basics."

In addition, in terms of diagnosis, might there be a difference between looking for the disease in the roots, or trunk, and looking for the root of the disease? And whose "trunk" are we even talking about? For an answer, let us return to the line as a whole in its present context. The specific meaning of the term *běn* 本 here is not as obvious as it might appear at first glance and has been subject to much scholarly and clinical debate. To give just two examples of how this line has been understood throughout history, it can refer to the six Qì 六氣 (the six climatic factors of Wind, Cold, Summerheat, Dampness, Dryness, and Fire), or to chronic, old conditions as opposed to newly emerging and passing "tip" (*biǎo* 標) manifestations. This is presumably how most modern practitioners of Chinese medicine understand this line when it is used out of context.

Many commentators on this particular chapter, however, do rightly emphasize the importance of the context and therefore the connection of the statement to the previous line and the chapter topic as a whole. I have attempted to do the same with my translation of *běn* as "the basics." As such, we might explain this "trunk" here as

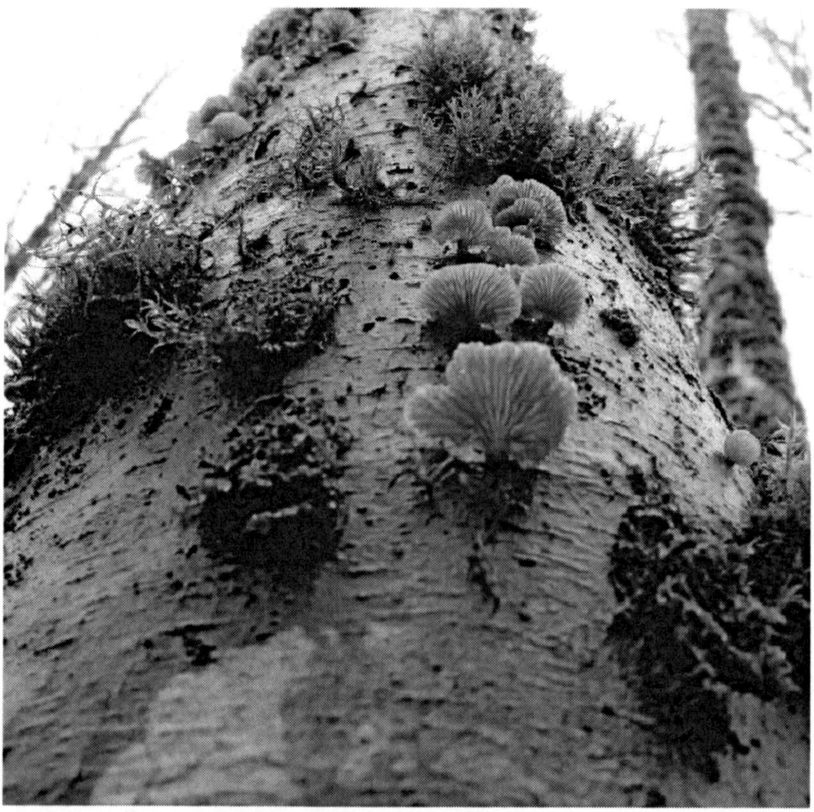

the foundation of all disease, which must be sought in the cosmic interplay of Yīn and Yáng. The Qīng-dynasty author Gāo Shìzōng 高士宗, for example, leaves no doubt on his reading of the line: "Where the *shén míng* resides, this then is the basis of [the disease in] Yīn and Yáng. Hence to treat disease, you must seek it in this basis" (神明所居，乃陰陽之本，故治病必求於本。). My reason for going into such detail here is that this line, in the present context, appears to go much further and entail much more than most modern Western practitioners are prepared to read into it. Rather than merely advising physicians to look for the root cause of symptoms in the body and address the underlying chronic conditions of imbalance instead of just the temporary manifestations of illness, this line reminds us of the need to study Yīn and Yáng as "the Dào of Heaven and Earth,... the guide ropes and connecting threads of the Myriad Things, the father and mother of Alterations and Transformations, the foundation and beginning of giving birth and taking life, and the Palace of the *shén míng*." In other words, this line sets the stage for connecting our pursuit of health in the human body with sagely insight into the macrocosmic dimensions of change through the prism of Yīn-Yáng dynamism as the Dào of Heaven and Earth. To prevent, diagnose, and treat disease in the body, whether our own as concerned individuals or that of our patients as professional healers, we must therefore cultivate our vision, our *míng* 明 in the sense of the ability to perceive the Dào, and learn to align ourselves and those around us as humans with the natural "Alterations and Transformations" between Heaven and Earth.

故積陽為天，積陰為地。
陰靜陽躁，陽生陰長，陽殺陰藏。

Gù jī yáng wéi tiān,
jī yīn wéi dì.
Yīn jìng yáng zào,
yáng shēng yīn zhǎng,
yáng shā yīn cáng.

Thus, accumulated Yáng
becomes Heaven;
accumulated Yīn becomes Earth.
Yīn stills and Yáng agitates;
Yáng gives life and
Yīn promotes growth;
Yáng takes life and
Yīn withdraws into storage.

Commentary by Gāo Shìzōng 高士宗

陰陽者，萬物之綱紀，故陰靜陽躁，靜而有常，
則為綱，躁而散殊，則為紀。

Yìn and Yáng are the guide ropes and connecting threads of the Myriad Things. As such, Yīn stills and Yáng agitates. When there is stillness, you have constancy. As a result, [Yīn can] serve as the guide ropes. When there is agitation, there is dispersal and diversification. As a result, [Yáng can] serve as the connecting threads.

The character *wéi* 為 can mean "to constitute" or "to serve/act/function as" or "to become," depending on context and the translator's preference. By necessity, an English translation has to pick one or the other of these possibilities since no equivalent word exists in English that can adequately express the full Chinese range of meanings in every context. Nevertheless, the reader should always keep in mind that all three of these meanings are possible and often implied, and that anybody can disagree with the translator's personal choice. Thus it would be just as correct to translate the line above as "...accumulated Yáng constitutes Heaven...." or "...accumulated Yáng functions as Heaven...."

Similarly, we can read *jìng* 靜 and *zào* 躁 either as verbs, as I have done above, or as adjectives, as "is still" and "is agitated." Regardless, when we tie this statement back to the first line of the chapter, as the Qīng period commentator Gāo Shìzōng has done, we can associate the stillness of Yīn with constancy (*cháng* 常) and thus with the "guide ropes" (*gāng* 綱), and the agitation of Yáng with diversification as expressed in the "connecting threads" (*jì* 紀) . At first glance, the English word "agitation," like the Chinese character *zào* 躁 that I have based my translation on, has the negative connotation of restlessness, impetuousness, rashness. Wiseman and Feng therefore define it as a technical medical term as "a subjective feeling of vexation outwardly expressed by pronounced abnormal movement."[11] It can, however, also be read as simply the opposite of stillness, the presence of movement. As so often in Chinese classical literature, we must be careful not to read value judgments into statements of complementarity. Here, the Daoist philosopher *Zhuāngzi* would ask us, who are we, with our limited perspective of frogs in a well, to know whether something is short or long, good or bad, black or white, dreaming or awakened reality, a butterfly or *Zhuāngzi*. The wording of this passage is a potent reminder that at least in early medical literature Yīn and Yáng are, with rare exceptions, complementary, equally important poles along a continuum of change, instead of the misogynistic expressions of an archaic and oppressive patriarchal and patrilineal society that values male over female, light over dark, white over black, activity over stillness, productivity over receptivity, and therefore Yáng over Yīn. As a matter of fact, early Chinese philosophical and self-cultivation literature like the *Nèi Yè* 內業 (Inward Training) quoted below tend to emphasize the need for stillness and quietude in order for humans to develop a stable heart, knowledgeable mind, and healthy body full of *jīng* Essence, Qì, and *Shén*.

* * *

Quotation from Nèi Yè 內業 (Inward Training)

天主正，地主平，人主安靜。

春秋冬夏，天之時也。山陵川谷，地之枝也。喜怒取予，人之謀也。

是故聖人與時變而不化，從物而不移，能正能靜，然後能定。

定心在中，耳目聰明，四枝堅固，可以為精舍。精也者，氣之精者也。

[11] Wiseman and Feng, 7.

Heaven rules correctness. Earth rules balance. Humanity rules peace and stillness.

Spring and autumn, winter and summer are the seasons of Heaven. Mountains and hills, rivers and valleys are the resources of Earth. Happiness and anger, taking and giving are the strategies of Humans.

For this reason, the sages alternate with the seasons but do not transform; follow along with things but do not shift position. Able to be correct, able to be still, then afterwards they are able to be stable.

With a stable heart in the center, the eyes and ears keenly perceptive, the four limbs firm and solid, they are able thereby to serve as an abode for Essence. This Essence! It is the Essence of Qì!

* * *

Like its often-quoted longer extrapolation "movement results in generating Yáng; stillness results in generating Yīn"(動則生陽；靜則生陰), this expression is important for medical treatments and such practices of health-cultivation or preventative medicine as qigong. In other words, if a patient is suffering from Yáng deficiency, increasing the level of physical activity may be a way to stimulate this aspect of their physiology. Anybody who has warmed up on a cold winter morning by going for a brisk walk is familiar with this simple truth. On the opposite spectrum, though, our modern capitalist lifestyle of constant productivity, pressure, rushing, and external excitement is causing a lot of patients to suffer from Yīn deficiency, which can be beautifully addressed by meditation or simply slowing down the pace of life and making conscious room for stillness. This advice may be particularly relevant for new (and old) mothers in the US who are often forced to juggle the demands of child-rearing with an intense professional life.

Especially in a cultural setting that overemphasizes the benefits of Yáng and values such aspects thereof as youth, expansion, activity, and productivity, this simple line here can serve as an important reminder to you and your patients to nourish and cultivate both Yáng and Yīn equally, and perhaps pay extra attention to signs of Yīn deficiency. We can see the problem of valuing Yáng over Yīn everywhere in our modern lifestyle, from women returning to work outside the home and pushing themselves too hard too soon after childbirth, to excessive exercise regimen by aging people in a sometimes ultimately unhealthy attempt to preserve the nubile bodies of our youth, to our addiction to devouring exciting and arousing news on TV, especially detrimental when done in the evening, and to the difficulty or reluctance to shift gears in the fall and winter to embrace the body's seasonal need for additional rest and quiet. This conundrum became particularly clear to me one winter when I was discussing the recommended activities laid out in *Sù Wèn* Chapter 2 on "Attuning the Spirit to the Four Qì" with a group of enthusiastic but overworked and sleep-deprived students.

* * *

Quotation from Sù Wèn[12]

冬三月，此謂閉藏，水冰地坼，無擾乎陽，早臥晚起，必待日光，
使志若伏若匿，若有私意，若已有得，去寒就溫，無泄皮膚使氣亟奪，
此冬氣之應，養藏之道也。逆之則傷腎，春為痿厥，奉生者少。

The three months of winter: This is the season referred to as "shuttering and storing." The water freezes and the earth cracks. Do not harass the Yáng and go to bed early and rise late! You must wait for the sunlight [to get up] and make your will appear as if lying low and going into hiding, as if having selfish intentions, as if having already obtained [something]. Avoid the cold and stay close to warmth, do not allow leakage through the skin and avoid extreme Qì deprivation. This is responding to the Qì of winter and the way of nurturing storage. If you go against it, you will injure the kidney. [As the result,] in spring [you will see] wilting and Reversal, and you will lack provisions to support sprouting.

[12] *Sù Wèn* 《素問》 Chapter 2, *Sì Qì Tiáo Shén Dà Lùn* 四氣調神大論 (Great Discourse on Attuning the Spirit to the Four Qì).

Implementing this advice in daily life within each of our personal, social, professional, and cultural constraints is, of course, not easy. But at least we can develop a sensitivity to the need for balance, which might allow us, over time, to develop a healthier and more sustainable lifestyle. In addition, we can also utilize this insight in the context of diagnosis: In clinic, we see that agitated patients are more likely to suffer from Yáng diseases, while still patients tend more towards Yīn conditions. And lastly, we can perhaps use this line of reasoning to explain the wonderful and well-documented calming and healing effect of water, the epitome of Yīn, on the human psyche.

The last phrase of this line, "Yáng gives life and Yīn promotes growth; Yáng takes life and Yīn withdraws into storage," is an interesting way to look at seasonal progression that differs from the more common association of the seasons with the Four—or Five if you include Earth,—dynamic agents: spring-Wood, summer-Fire, autumn-Metal, and winter-Water. As *Sù Wèn* Chapter 2 lays out in detail and many other texts support, the four seasons are most often associated with the terms *sheng* 生 "sprouting/birth" for spring, *zhǎng* 長 "growth" for summer, *shōu* 收 "harvest/receive" for autumn, and *cáng* 藏 "storage" for winter. In addition, spring and summer are usually associated with the Yáng half of the year, with increasing warmth, activity, expansion, and outward direction, while autumn and winter are considered the time when Yīn prevails, a time for slowing down, gathering in, and turning inward, for receptivity, restraint, and contraction. Replacing *shōu* "harvest/receiving" with *shā* 殺 "taking life" for the activity associated with autumn is a minor change that makes perfect sense. Autumn is, after all, the season for going on military expeditions and meting out punishments, in the spirit of the first killing frosts of the season that harshly end the growth and abundance of summer. I should also clarify that the word "withdraw" here is used in the transitive sense of acting on a direct object, of removing something by putting it into storage. More importantly and surprisingly, though, the associations of Yīn with *zhǎng* 長 "growth" and thereby indirectly with summer and fire, and of Yáng with *shā* 殺 "taking life" and hence with autumn and metal, contrast sharply with our customary understanding of these two seasons. The descriptions of these two seasons in *Sù Wèn* Chapter 2 leave no doubt in mind that summer there falls into the Yáng half of the year and autumn into the Yīn half. Zhāng Zhìcōng 張志聰 offers an elegant attempt at an explanation: "Spring and summer are the Yīn and Yáng of Heaven, and [Heaven] thus governs Yáng['s function of] giving life and Yīn['s function of] promoting growth. Autumn and winter are the Yīn and Yáng of Earth, and [Earth] thus governs Yáng['s function of] taking life and Yīn['s function of withdrawing into storage" (春夏者。天之陰陽也。故主陽生陰長。秋冬者。地之陰陽也。故主陽殺陰藏。).

I leave it to you, dear reader, to grapple with this contradiction on your own, and suggest that you embrace this situation as a common theme in this chapter that we will return to again and again: the ever-deepening complexity of the interplay between Yīn and Yáng as we detect aspects of one nestled within the other within the other within the other, and so on *ad infinitum*. Perhaps, in future years, this line will help you appreciate a different aspect as you experience summer growth and autumn harvest in a more balanced way by embracing the Yīn within the Yáng (in the case of summer) and the Yáng within the Yīn (in the case of autumn).

* * *

Quotation from Sù Wèn[13]

夏三月，此謂蕃秀，天地氣交，萬物華實，夜臥早起，無厭於日，使志無怒，使華英成秀，使氣得泄，若所愛在外，此夏氣之應，養長之道也。。。。

秋三月，此謂容平，天氣以急，地氣以明，早臥早起，與雞俱興，使志安寧，以緩秋刑，收斂神氣，使秋氣平，無外其志，使肺氣清，此秋氣之應，養收之道也。

The three months of summer: This is [the season] referred to as "thriving and bursting into full bloom." The Qì of Heaven and Earth intermingle, and the Myriad Things form flowers and fruit. Go to bed [late] at night and rise early! Do not get indolent during the day and do not let your will be affected by anger! Make it flourish and bear fruit, and allow the Qì to spill out, as if what you love is on the outside. This is responding to the Qì of summer and the way of nurturing growth.

The three months of autumn: This is the season referred to as "receiving and balance." The Qì of heaven thereby is harsh and the Qì of earth thereby is clear. Go to bed early and rise early, stirring with the chickens! Let your will be calm and tranquil, in order to relax the punishments of autumn! Gather in and restrain your spirit and your Qì, to make the Qì of autumn balanced. Do not allow your will to stray outside and thereby make your lung Qì clear. This is responding to the Qì of autumn and the way of nurturing harvest.

* * *

[13] *Sù Wèn* 《素問》 Chapter 2.

陽化氣，陰成形。

Yáng huà Qì,
yīn chéng xíng.

Yáng creates Qì;
Yīn completes the Form.

Commentary by Zhāng Zhìcōng 張志聰[14]

天主生物，地主成物。故陽化萬物之氣，而吾人之氣，由陽化之。陰成萬物之形，而吾人之形，由陰成之。

Heaven is in charge of engendering things; Earth is in charge of completing things. As such, Yáng creates the Qì of the Myriad Things, and the Qì of us humans is [also] created by Yáng. Yīn completes the Form of the Myriad Things, and the Form of us humans is [also] completed by Yīn.

NO BOOK ON EARLY CHINESE MEDICAL LITERATURE CAN DELVE VERY deeply into the subject before having to address the thorny issue of how to define and conceptualize the early Chinese equivalent of what we in English tend to call the "body." What is it that these texts are talking about, and what are its parameters? Following the theme of this book, the present line suggests a dualistic approach, namely the juxtaposition of Qì, associated with Yáng, and *xíng* 形 (below translated as "form"), associated with Yīn. Now it is tempting to simply superimpose our Western and biomedical Cartesian split between the material and the immaterial realm on this line, call it "energy" and "matter," or "energetic body" and "material body," and move on. I wish it were that easy! Discussions on the nature and properties of Qì have been ongoing in the West already for decades, with whole books written on the subject, so there is no need to reinvent the wheel and regurgitate old arguments. As anybody with basic training in Chinese medicine, philosophy, science, or literary language knows, equating Qì with "energy" or "breath" or the "immaterial realm" quickly becomes an obstacle to an accurate understanding of the concept in

[14] Zhāng Zhìcōng 《張志聰》, *Huáng Dì Nèi Jīng Sù Wèn Jí Zhù* 黃帝內經素問集注 (Collected Commentaries on the Yellow Emperor's Inner Classic: Plain Questions, 1670).

the vast majority of contexts. Qì is simply Qì, with no English word that can possibly serve as an equivalent. For the purposes of the present book I am comfortable leaving it at that and trusting that my readers know what it is, based on their felt experiences and clinical training. Unfortunately, the term *xíng* is much less familiar to most Western practitioners of Chinese medicine and therefore requires an explanation. And again unfortunately, it is as misleading to equate *xíng* with matter or the material body as it is to equate Qì with energy. Then what is it, and what is the meaning of the statement, "Yáng catalyzes the formation of Qì; Yīn completes the *xing*"?

In contrast to the translation of *xíng* by Unschuld and Tessenow as "physical appearance," I follow Rochat de la Vallée in translating the term as "form" for reasons that will become apparent below.[15] In her article on "Outward Form (xing 形) and Inward Qi 氣: The 'Sentimental Body' in Early Chinese Medicine," the anthropologist Elisabeth Hsu offers important insights. In Warring States and early Hàn literature like the Zhāngjiāshān 張家山 and Mǎwángduī 馬王堆 manuscripts, the above-mentioned *Nèi Yè* 內業 (Inner Cultivation), and early textual layers of the *Nèi Jīng*, Hsu detects a dualistic conception of a "sentimental body" of a Yīn-Yáng, up-down, and inward-outward dynamic. She contrasts this dualistic "sentimental body," developed with the aim of regulating individual emotions, with what she calls the "body ecologic." This is a later pentic view that envisions a five-fold conception of the body on the basis of the Five *Zàng* 藏 organs, stresses the seasonality of illness, and was perhaps developed in response to the needs of the Hàn imperial administration to manage not individual bodies but large populations and their prevailing disorders. According to Hsu, the dual body of inner Qì and outer form is one whose external aspect can be examined visually and therefore diagnosed by the trained observer, especially for fullness or emptiness in the vessels and in terms of color. This external aspect of the "form" is associated, in health and illness, with external forces like the pathogenic seasonal factors. As Hsu explains, "…this outwardly visible body contrasted with body-internal aspects that could not be

[15] Unschuld and Tessenow, 96; Rochat de la Vallée, 13.

apprehended through vision directly, such as the emotions and feelings, the will, one's spirits and qi."[16] In this pairing of inner Qì and outer form, Hsu makes a convincing case that Qì here refers not to an external atmospheric substance to be inhaled, consumed, collected, and concentrated inside the human body but "can be seen to allude to body-internal processes such as thought and sentiment."[17]

* * *

Quotation from the Nèi Yè 《內業》

凡人之生也，天出其精，地出其形，合此以為人；和乃生，不和不生。

In the lives of all humans, Heaven brings forth the Essence, and Earth brings forth the Form. By matching these two up, humanity exists. Harmony means life; absence of harmony means absence of life.

* * *

The next thorny issue that needs to be addressed is the meaning of the character *huà* 化, which I have decided, after much hesitation, to translate as "to create" in the above line. Directly related to whether we interpret *huà*, as is customarily done and quite appropriate in many contexts, as "transform" or, as I suggest here, as "create," the key question then becomes this: Is Qì, in the present context, a substance that is engendered inside the body through the involvement of Yáng, or is it an external substance that is drawn into the body from the atmospheric environment, as more contemporary accounts of Chinese medicine tend to suggest? Is it something that is available universally in unlimited amounts and merely needs to be condensed or otherwise processed to become something tangible, perceptible, useful for nourishing the human body, or is it a substance

[16] Hsu, *Outward Form and Inward Qi,* 119.

[17] Ibid., 121.

that is generated by and inside the individual? The serious ramifications of one's answer for physical cultivation and medical practice are obvious. Unfortunately, *huà* is simply a concept that has no equivalent in English, and no translation can fully encompass its meaning. Suffice it to say that Yáng is associated with Qì as the internal aspect of the body in an action that initiates change, while Yīn is associated with Form as the external aspect of the body in an action that completes change.

From a medical perspective, we can follow Dr. Long Rihui's lead and interpret this passage as follows: Yáng acts on Qì by dispersing *wèi qì* (defense Qì), while Yīn completes the Form, here in the sense of the material aspects or containing elements of the body, such as *jīng* Essence, Blood, flesh, and other Yīn materials. In treatment, we use warming medicinals to tonify Yáng and thereby stimulate the body's defense. Cases of Yīn deficiency mean that the material aspect of the body is incomplete, as in congenital deficiencies in newborn babies, which should be treated with formulas like Liù Wèi Dìhuáng Wán 六味地黄丸.

寒極生熱，熱極生寒。寒氣生濁，熱氣生清。
清氣在下，則生飧泄；濁氣在上，則生䐜脹。
此陰陽反作，病之逆從也。

Hán jí shēng rè, rè jí shēng hán.
Hán qì shēng zhuó, rè qì shēng qīng.
Qīng qì zài xià, zé shēng sūn xiè;
zhuó qì zài shàng, zé shēng chēn zhàng.

Cǐ yīn yáng fǎn zuò, bìng zhī nì cóng yě.

Extremes of Cold engender Heat; extremes of Heat engender Cold. Cold Qì engenders turbidity; Heat Qì engenders clearness. When clear Qì is located below, it engenders diarrhea with undigested food particles; when turbid Qì is located above, it engenders swelling and distention.

These are the contrary actions of Yīn and Yáng, and the manifestations of disease that go against the proper course of things.

With this passage, we finally enter a section of the text that is clearly intended to explain processes inside the human body. The first sentence is often read as referring to the phenomenon of False Heat or Warmth, a process whereby Yáng that is getting pushed up and out can temporarily cause superficial heat as the result of an underlying extreme deep internal Cold condition. This process leads to such outward manifestations of Heat as a hot head or flushed cheeks. As the text continues, the opposite situation is also possible, namely the body's response to an underlying extreme Heat condition by manifesting Cold symptoms on the outside. An alternative clinical interpretation of this line would be a Yángmíng Fǔ syndrome where Heat is locked inside but cannot effuse to the outside, causing false Cold symptoms in the exterior.

According to Dr. Long, however, the first sentence should be read as referring to diseases in their critical stage. Since such cases are nowadays generally addressed in the emergency room of your local biomedical hospital rather than in the acupuncturist's office, modern practitioners of Chinese medicine may not be as familiar with this situation. To name just two examples, we see lots of chills and cold symptoms in the initial stages of malaria, but these turn into fever and other increasingly severe Heat symptoms when the disease reaches a critical stage. Similarly, in babies with severe high temperatures, we see the body turning cold.

When we apply the same phrase to the natural world, which may help us understand the expression of this situation in the human body, the alternating changes of Yīn and Yáng are easily measurable and observable. During the three 15-day seasonal nodes that follow the summer and winter solstices, namely *xiàzhì* 夏至 (summer solstice), *xiǎoshǔ* 小暑 (small heat), and *dàshǔ* 大暑 (great heat) and *dōngzhì* 冬至 (winter solstice),*xiǎohán* 小寒 (small cold), and *dàhán* 大寒 (great cold), the foundations are laid for the reversal of weather and the return of cold or heat thereafter. As this example shows, it is important that we read Yīn and Yáng first as laws of nature and only secondly as a philosophy. As a third step, we can then interpret them as medical concepts that demonstrate the concrete applications of the

Dào of nature at the site of the human body, to be experienced directly and personally.

Another way in which I personally have experienced the truth of this line is with my daily swim in the Salish Sea. The water being around 48°F, or just shy of 9°C, for most of the year, the experience might not quite qualify as "extreme of cold" but still can give me a taste of this heat-cold dynamic. After just a few seconds of being immersed in the icy water, the initial feeling of cold completely disappears as my body adjusts to the cold. Coming out of the water at the end of my swim, before I eventually start shivering, I always experience invigorating surges of hot blood penetrating into every nook and cranny of my being.

Turning now to the descriptions of pathology in this passage, in a healthy person Heat from the Spleen and Stomach causes clear Qì to ascend to the Lung and facilitate the sprinkler function of the Lung there, while turbid Qì is supposed to descend. When this direction is reversed so that clear Qì descends into the lower body instead, this indicates pathology, manifesting in diarrhea. To facilitate diagnostic specificity, the text elaborates that the particular diarrhea witnessed in this circumstance is one of "diarrhea with undigested food particles" (*sūn xiè* 飧泄). The character *sūn* can mean "supper" but originally means to soak rice in water to prepare it for cooking. Here, most commentators agree that it refers to a type of diarrhea that looks like *sūn*, or in other words an outpouring of only partially digested food. This symptom indicates a weakening and dropping of center Qì, manifesting in inadequate functioning of the Spleen and Stomach. As the result, these organs fail to extract the Subtle Essences (*jīngwēi* 精微) from food and drink and transport them to the upper body, instead eliminating them in the stool. An often-cited alternative reading suggested by the *Shèng Jì Zǒng Lù* 《聖濟總錄》 (Comprehensive Record of the sage's Rescue) is based on the etymology of the character 飧, a combination of "evening" 夕 with "food" 食. This text would suggest a translation of *sūn xiè* as "dinnertime diarrhea," and can also be justified clinically since evening is the time when meals are particularly hard to transform and hence a likely time for the elimination of undigested food.

The presence of turbid Qì in the upper body, on the other hand, is described by the term *chēn zhàng* 瞋脹. Both of these characters refer to an inflated, bloated appearance, usually explained as an indication of impaired Lung function and resulting accumulation of fluids. The *Lèi Jīng* hence explains this compound as "fullness in the chest and diaphragm." Here, we can relate this symptom to turbid Qì rising, due to the inability of the intestines to push food down to the rectum. Instead of being expelled, it ascends to the Middle *Jiāo* and causes congestion in the rib-sides and chest. For these kinds of conditions, Lǐ Dōngyuán's 李東垣 focus on promoting the raising of clear Yáng Qì by regulating the Spleen and Stomach and thereby causing turbid Yīn Qì to descend naturally may be an ideal choice. Bǔ Zhōng Yì Qì Tāng 補中益氣湯 represents this treatment approach. Another option for babies or seniors with digestive issues may be Shēn Líng Báizhú Sǎn 參苓白朮散. Qì-moving prescriptions, on the other hand, may aggravate such conditions instead of strengthening the Spleen and Stomach.

While the general meaning of the second part of this passage is fairly straightforward, a brief note on grammar may be helpful for readers with some background in classical Chinese. According to most commentators, *fǎn* 反 here should be interpreted as *fān* 翻, to turn something upside down, causing a state that is the opposite of what it is supposed to be like. The two characters *nì cóng* 逆從 can be interpreted in three different ways: First, we can read them in accordance with the *Lèi Jīng* as a pair of verbs that describe movement in opposite directions, namely "going against the flow" (in the sense of *fǎn* 反) and "following along" (in the sense of *shùn* 順). Second, we can read them also as a pair of verbs but with a different meaning, as "welcoming and sending off." To support this usage, see *Líng Shū* 靈樞 Chapter 1, there referring to the movement of the Blood and Qì in the vessels and the physician's response in treatment. As a third option, we can follow Wú Kūn 吳崑 and read them as a Verb-Object combination in the sense of "going against what is proper or healthy," with *nì* 逆 being parallel to *fǎn* 反in the previous phrase.

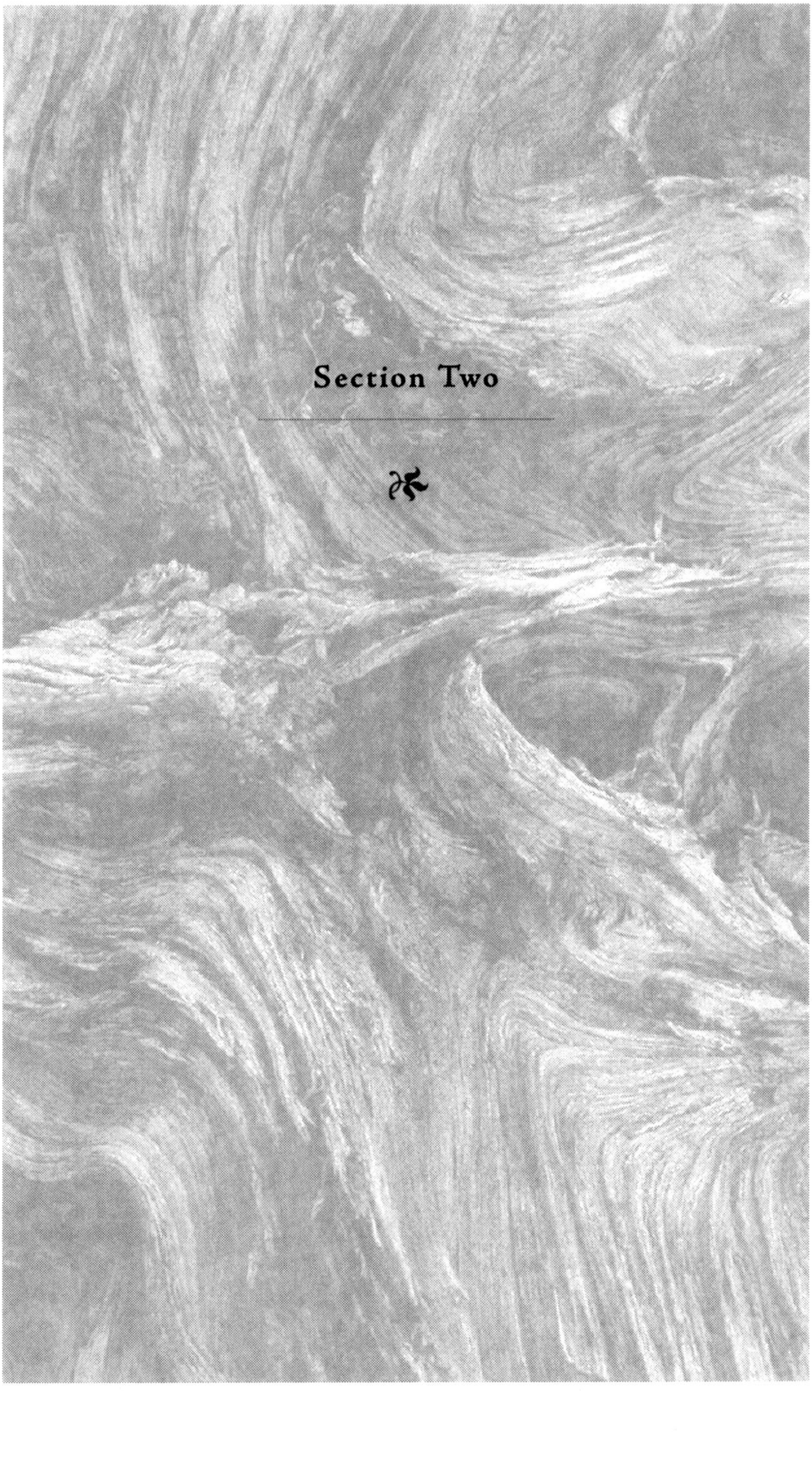

Section Two

故清陽為天，濁陰為地；地氣上為雲，天氣下為雨；雨出地氣，雲出天氣。

Gù qīng yáng wéi tiān,
zhuó yīn wéi dì; dì qì shàng
wéi yún, tiān qì xià wéi yǔ; yǔ
chū dì qì, yún chū tiān qì.

Therefore, clear Yáng constitutes Heaven; turbid Yīn constitutes Earth. Earth Qì, rising up, becomes clouds; Heaven Qì, coming down, becomes rain. Rain emanates from Earth Qì; clouds emanate from Heaven Qì.

In general, Yáng rises up to Heaven while Yīn descends down to Earth. As such, it is the logical result that accumulated Yáng is associated with Heaven, and accumulated Yīn with Earth. Nevertheless, any separation between Yīn and Yáng, whether in the body or in nature, will lead to disorder and pathology, and eventually to death. The present line hence describes the healthy ideal state of continuous interaction and connection between Yīn and Yáng, which results from the fact that the process reverses direction as soon as it has reached its peak. Yáng Qì, coming out of the Earth, has thus ascended to its extreme in the form of clouds, which represents Yīn reaching up to Yáng. This Qì then reverses direction and descends as rain, connecting back down to Yīn. When Yīn Qì, emanating from Heaven, has descended to its lowest state in the form of rain that has fallen back down onto the Earth, thereby connecting Yáng down to Yīn, it has to turn around to rise from the Earth as clouds, connecting back up with Yáng. In other words, clouds rise up and up and up in a Yáng process until they reach a layer of cold that forces them to precipitate down as Yīn rain. This moisture falls onto the warm Earth, becomes absorbed, and then, under the influence of heat from the sun or the hot surface, evaporates to rise, starting the process anew in a never-ending cycle. We can thus interpret the term "emanate from" here in the sense of "is rooted in." As the Qīng-period commentator Zhāng Zhìcōng explains, "Yīn Qì and Yáng Qì rise up and sink down to interact with each other. Afterwards, the clouds move and the rain bestows, thereby creating the Myriad Things (陰陽之氣，上下相交，然後雲行雨施，而化生萬物也。)."

Living in the rainforest of the Pacific Northwest, the interaction between Yīn and Yáng through the intermingling of clouds and rain is not hard to visualize. It surely makes intuitive sense that Yáng, being clear, light, and diffuse, rises up to Heaven, while Yīn, being murky, dark, and dense, sinks down to Earth. Heaven and Earth are, after all, the primary referents that this text uses over and over to help us conceptualize the actions and reactions of these two basic forces of the universe. I have two images that come to my mind to illustrate these statements: On the one hand, visualize a warm spring day where the new sun shines down with all its radiant vigor onto the dark rich damp soil of a freshly tilled field. As a result, we literally see clouds rising in the form of steam. Perhaps this scene is made even more dramatic by fog slowly rising from the valley below, engulfing us for moments or hours, to finally reveal the clear blue morning sky when the fog has passed. To visualize Yīn sinking down, I can picture myself in the middle of a thick Oregon rainforest on one of those grey drizzly soupy winter days. There is so much moisture in the air that the minuscule droplets almost hang suspended in the air and collect on every tiny surface that catches them, rather than falling straight down. The verdant lushness, seemingly eternal presence, and resilience of the old growth forest around me, with infinitesimal numbers of plants and animals growing and decaying and reproducing on every inch of surface is fueled and nourished by the moisture falling from the sky as Heaven's Qì for months on end.

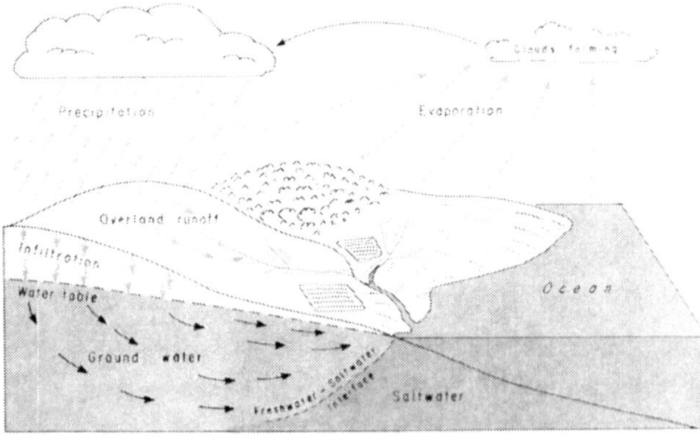

Water Cycle

What is perhaps harder to understand is how rain, identified as Heaven Qì coming down, then "emanates from Earth Qì" and how clouds, identified as Earth Qì rising up, "emanate from Heaven Qì." I am not sure whether the Yellow Emperor had in mind the complex meteorological processes of evaporation, condensation, and precipitation demonstrated in this illustration of the water cycle, or whether he simply observed that rain falls out of clouds, which are Earth Qì that has risen up, while clouds rise out of soil wetted by rain, which is Heaven Qì that has fallen.

In the end, this statement serves as a reminder of perhaps the single most central message of this entire text: the need for Yīn and Yáng to interact, to complement each other, to engage in a never-ending circle of sinking and rising apart until they reach the extreme and then reversing direction and coming together, only to start the process anew. As humans in the Yellow Emperor's world, we are the link between Heaven and Earth, between Yīn and Yáng, in our personal, social, and professional lives (whether as farmers, healers, or rulers), and therefore can play an important role in restoring the dynamic equilibrium between these two opposite yet complementary forces. Separation means death, engagement means life. It really is that simple.

* * *

Commentary by Zhāng Zhìcōng 張志聰

地雖在下，而地氣上升為雲。天雖在上，而天氣下降為雨。
夫由雲而後有雨，是雨雖天降，而實本地氣所升之雲，故云出地氣。
由雨之降，而後有雲之升，是雲雖地升，而實本天氣所降之雨。故云出天氣。
此陰陽交互之道也，而人亦應之。此篇言天地之陰陽，與人之陰陽相合。
是以一節言天地陰陽水火，一節言清濁臟腑精形，以天人相間而言也。

Even though Earth is below, Earth Qì rises to become clouds. Even though Heaven is above, Heaven Qì descends to become rain. Now the reason why we have rain after clouds is that even though rain is Heaven descending, in actuality it is based in the clouds that are the rising of Earth Qì. For this reason, we say that "it emanates from Earth Qì." The reason why we have clouds rising after a rainfall is that even though clouds are Earth rising, in actually they are based in the rain that is the falling down of Heaven Qì. For this reason, we say that "they emanate from Heaven Qì." This is the Dào of Yīn and Yáng intermingling with each other, and humans also resonate with this. This chapter talks about the fact that Yīn and Yáng of Heaven and Earth match up with Yīn and Yáng in humans. As such, one section talks about Heaven and Earth, Yīn and Yáng, and fire and water, and another section talks about the clear and the turbid, the zàng and Fǔ Organs, and Essence and Form, thereby alternatingly talking about Heaven and Humanity.

故清陽出上竅，濁陰出下竅；清陽發腠理，濁陰走五臟；清陽實四肢，濁陰歸六腑。

Gù qīng yáng chū shàng qiào, zhuó yīn chū xià qiào; qīng yáng fā còu lǐ, zhuó yīn zǒu wǔ zàng; qīng yáng shí sì zhī, zhuó yīn guī liù fǔ.

Therefore, clear Yáng exits from the upper apertures; turbid Yīn exits from the lower apertures. Clear Yáng disperses outward through the texture lines of the skin and flesh; turbid Yīn runs into the Five Zàng Organs. Clear Yáng fills the four extremities; turbid Yīn homes to the Six Fǔ Organs.

Commentary by Wáng Bīng 王冰[1]

氣本乎天者親上，氣本乎地者親下，各從其類也。上竅，謂耳目鼻口。下竅，謂前陰後陰。

The reason why Qì that is based in Heaven has an affinity to the upper body and why Qì that is based in Earth has an affinity to the lower body, is that each accords with its category. The "upper apertures" refers to the ears, eyes, nostrils, and mouth; the "lower apertures" refers to the genitals and anus.

Perhaps by intentionally employing specific technical terminology in this line, the authors make it clear that they are now applying the general guidelines and observations from the previous statement to the concrete microcosm of the human body: The term *qiào* 竅, translated above as "apertures," does not pose many problems and has been explained throughout history as "caves" (*xué* 穴) or "holes" (*kǒng* 孔). In the context of the human body, the "nine apertures" are consistently defined as seven in the upper body, associated with Yáng, and two in the lower body, associated with Yīn. This definition still holds true in modern TCM, as reflected in Wiseman and Feng's translation as "orifice" and their explanation: "Any of the openings of the body. The *upper orifices* or *clear orifices* are the eyes, ears, nostrils, mouth, and tongue, whereas the *lower orifices* or *turbid orifices* are the anal and genital orifices. These are collectively referred to as the *nine orifices.*"[2]

The next technical term, "texture lines of the skin and flesh," is my translation for *còulǐ* 腠理. Rendered as "interstices" by Wiseman and left untranslated by other translators, this term has been explained in historical sources as the lines or striations in the flesh below, and

[1] Wáng Bīng 王冰 is the original commentator of the *Nèi Jīng* from the Táng dynasty.

[2] Wiseman and Feng, *Practical Dictionary,* 421.

possibly including, the skin. In either case, the earliest transmitted written record is found in Biǎn Què's 扁鵲 biography in the *Shǐ Jì* 史記 (Historian's Records). In that text, it refers to the superficial texture in the flesh, a location for disease where it is still easy to treat. The *Shǐ jì* line reads: "The lord has an illness located in the *còulǐ*, which if left untreated, will go deeper."

Quotation from the Shǐ Jì 史記[3]

扁鵲過齊，齊桓侯客之。入朝見，曰：「君有疾在腠理，不治將深。」桓侯曰：「寡人無疾。」扁鵲出，桓侯謂左右曰：「醫之好利也，欲以不疾者為功。」

後五日，扁鵲復見，曰：「君有疾在血脈，不治恐深。」桓侯曰：「寡人無疾。」扁鵲出，桓侯不悅。

後五日，扁鵲復見，曰；「君有疾在腸胃閒，不治將深。」桓侯不應。扁鵲出，桓侯不悅。

後五日，扁鵲復見，望見桓侯而退走。桓侯使人問其故。扁鵲曰：「疾之居腠理也，湯熨之所及也；在血脈，鍼石之所及也；其在腸胃，酒醪之所及也；其在骨髓，雖司命無柰之何。今在骨髓，臣是以無請也。」

後五日，桓侯體病，使人召扁鵲，扁鵲已逃去。桓侯遂死。

When Biǎn Què was passing through Qí, Duke Huán invited him. Entering the audience, Biǎn Què said: "Your majesty has an illness in the texture lines of the flesh and skin. If left untreated, it is about to go deeper." Duke Huán replied: "We do not have an illness." Biǎn Què exited, and Duke Huán commented to his attendants: "This is a physician's love of profit. He wants to exploit a situation with somebody who is not sick."

[3] Biography of Biǎn Què in Sīmǎ Qiān 《司馬遷》、*Shǐ Jì* 史記 (Records of the Historian).

After five days, Biǎn Què returned for an audience and said: "Your majesty has an illness in the blood vessels. If left untreated, I fear that it will go deeper." Duke Huán responded: "We do not have an illness." Biǎn Què exited, and Duke Huán was not happy.

After five more days, Biǎn Què again returned for an audience and said: "Your majesty has an illness in the area of the intestines and stomach. If left untreated, it is about to go deeper." Duke Huán did not respond. Biǎn Què exited, and Duke Huán was not happy.

After fiver more days, Biǎn Què again returned for an audience. Seeing Duke Huán in the distance, he retreated and left. Duke Huán sent somebody to ask for the reason. Biǎn Què answered: "When the disease was residing in the texture lines of the flesh and skin, it could have been reached with hot liquids and hot compresses. When the disease was residing in the blood vessels, it could have been reached with needles and stones. When it was in the intestines and stomach, it could have been reached with medicinal liquors and wines. But once it is in the bones and marrow, not even the Divine Commander of Destiny can do anything about it. Now that your disease is in the bones and marrow, your servant therefore has no reason to pay you his respects."

After five more days, Duke Huán's body fell ill, and he sent a person to summon Biǎn Què. But Biǎn Què had already fled away. Duke Huán consequently died.

* * *

In a little more medical detail, the *Jīn Guì Yào Lüè* 金匱要略 (Essential Prescriptions from the Golden Cabinet) explains: "*Còu* is the location where the Triple *Jiāo* meets up with and connects to the true source, where the Blood and Qì pour into. *Lǐ* are the patterns in the skin and *zàngfǔ* organs" (腠者，是三焦通會元真之處，為血氣所注。理者，是皮膚臟腑之文理也。). In clinical practice, it is perhaps easiest to think of the *còulǐ* as structures in the space between the skin and the flesh, somewhat overlapping but not identical with the biomedical concept of subcutaneous fascia.

Lastly, a note may be necessary to explain the meaning of turbid Yīn "homing" to the Six *Fǔ* Organs. "Home" is my translation for the character *guī* 歸. In the Hàn dynasty dictionary *Shuō Wén Jiě Zì* 說文解字 (Explaining Graphs and Elucidating Characters), this character is defined as a woman getting married (hence the etymology of a foot, a wall, and a broom). The character is most commonly translated as "to return." The connection between these two concepts may require some explaining for Western readers: In traditional Chinese patrilineal society, daughters were raised with the clear awareness that they would eventually leave their natal family to become a part of the husband's clan. Regardless of emotional ties, regional and economic variations, and complications in real life, the ideal society, at least the imagination of the literate elite, which was the segment of society that created the written language, was one in which a woman's ultimate resting place, her final destination in life, and hence her "home," was not her natal family but her husband's family. As such, the character has the connotation of arriving at the place where a person or thing belongs, rather than of returning to a place where somebody or something has been before. *Guī* can also be used in the sense of a person who is withdrawing from society to the mountains, usually at the end of a busy social life, to arrive at his or her true destination, which is a place of rest and refuge. Following Wiseman and Feng, I have chosen to translate it as "to home to" as an active verb, in the sense of "call something home" or "make something home." In many contexts, you could be justified in reading it in the sense of "to be associated with" (*shǔ yú* 屬於). I follow Wiseman's choice here because it does work in the present context to adequately convey this sense of movement to the place where a person or substance belongs. As the etymology cited above suggests, the more elegant "to return to" is too narrow in English and therefore potentially misleading in the context of this text here and in the following section.

Looking at this entire section in clinical terms, "clear Yáng" refers to the Yáng Qì that nourishes the sense organs (exits from the upper apertures), disperses outward through the exterior layer of the body, and warms and animates the body, creating vitality by filling the four limbs and enabling smooth movements and strength through healthy motor functions. As *wèiqì* (defense Qì), this clear Yáng controls the opening and closing of the orifices in the skin and the body's defense to the outside. Turbid Yīn can be read as a reference to Essence and Blood, as extracted from food and drink, which move into and are stored in the Five *Zàng* Organs, while the waste products are processed through the Six *Fǔ* Organs to be eliminated as feces and urine through the lower orifices.

* * *

Commentary by Zhāng Zhìcōng 張志聰

人之清陽本乎天而出上竅。人之濁陰本乎地而出下竅。言人之陰陽猶雲之升，雨之降，通乎天地之氣也。

The clear Yáng of human beings is rooted in Heaven and thus exits from the upper apertures. The turbid Yīn of human beings is rooted in Earth and thus exits from the lower orifices. This is saying that the Yīn and Yáng of humans is like the ascending movement of clouds and the descending movement or rain, connecting with the Qì of Heaven and Earth.

* * *

水為陰，火為陽；陽為氣，陰為味。

Shuǐ wéi yīn, huǒ wéi yáng;
yáng wéi qì, yīn wéi wèi.

Water is Yīn; Fire is Yáng.
Yáng is Qì; Yīn is Flavor.

Commentary by Gāo Shìzōng 高士宗

在天為寒，在地為水，故水為陰。在天為熱，在地為火，故火為陽。陽主輕清，故陽為氣，陰主重濁，故陰為味。

[Yīn] in Heaven constitutes Cold and on Earth constitutes Water, hence Water is Yīn. [Yáng] in Heaven constitutes Heat and on Earth constitutes Fire, hence Fire is Yáng. Yáng rules what is light and clear, hence Yáng constitutes Qì. Yīn rules what is heavy and turbid, hence Yīn constitutes Flavor.

Commentary by Zhāng Jièbīn 張介賓

故天以日月為水火，易以坎離為水火，醫以心腎為水火，丹以精氣為水火。夫腎者水也，水中生氣，即真火也；心者火也，火中生液，即真水也。水火互藏，乃至道之所在，醫家首宜省察。

Thus in Heaven, the sun and moon are Water and Fire; in the Yì Jīng, [the trigrams] kǎn and lí are Water and Fire; in medicine, the Heart and the Kidney are Water and Fire; and in alchemy, Essence and Qì are Water and Fire. Now the Kidney is Water, and the creation of Qì inside Water is precisely True Fire; the Heart is Fire, and the creation of fluids inside Fire is precisely True Water. The mutual storage of Water and Fire within each other, this is where the ultimate Dào is located, and this is what any physician should first examine attentively.

The commentary on this line from Zhāng Jièbīn's *Lèi Jīng*, which was published in 1624, is interesting to me for a number of reasons. Of course we should never consider an interpretation that is more than a thousand years removed from the original compilation of the *Nèi Jīng* as authoritative or the only possible reading. Nevertheless, we can learn a lot about historical Chinese medicine from these sorts of comments, especially if we contextualize them with similar literature from the same time period.

First, what this passage shows us is unfortunately not how the original authors, compilers, and readers of the *Nèi Jīng* understood this line and read the *Nèi Jīng* as a whole. Nevertheless, we can get a glimpse of how physicians and medical authors in the late Míng period approached and contemplated such seemingly simple short passages as "Water is Yīn; Fire is Yáng." As such, Fire and Water (and thus by implication Yáng and Yīn) are here read in the following contexts: in astronomy as sun and moon; in cosmology, couched in the language of the *Yì Jīng* 易經 (Classic of Changes), as the two basic trigrams *kǎn* ☵ and *lí* ☲ (Water as a solid Yáng line enclosed by two broken Yīn lines, and Fire as a broken Yīn line enclosed by two solid Yáng lines); in medicine as the two *zàng* organs Heart and Kidney; and in alchemy as the precious substances Qì and Essence, respectively.

The art of the physician, like the arts of the philosopher, cosmologist, astronomer, diviner, and alchemist, can thus be said to be encapsulated in this ability to transcend realms, or microcosmic perspectives, and to grasp the multiple microcosmic dimensions of any situation, to thereby plumb its meaning more fully and ultimately from a macrocosmic perspective, sages or "seers" are able to access the associations and experiences they might have in any one of these contexts and relate them to all the other contexts. Thereby they can shed light for themselves and others on this interaction of the two most basic forces of life, Yīn and Yáng, Water and Fire, and then apply this insight to any context and microcosm, from politics to agriculture to medicine, and to internal and external alchemy. Understanding the life-giving dance between these two foundational elements in the cosmos is the cornerstone of the sage's ability to decipher the sky and make calendric predictions in astronomy, to assess a given situation by means of the 64 hexagrams of the *Yì Jīng* and predict future potentials and risks in divination, to diagnose and treat illness in medicine, and to cultivate oneself for longevity and ultimately achieve transcendence of the restraints of the human body in alchemy.

What all these skills have in common is the ability to understand the direction of change from that which has already manifested to that which has not manifested yet. Seeing the seed of invisible future developments by accurately assessing the visible present in light of the direction and dynamic of past changes allows the sage to position him- or herself in alignment with the Dào, to act in a manner that is *shùn* 順 (following along with the currents) instead of *nì* 逆 (going against the current). Two modern equivalents of this skill may be to ride the waves of change like a skilled surfer or to plant in harmony with short- and long-term celestial cycles as an experienced biodynamic farmer.

In a physician, an expression of this skill can be found in the choice of therapeutic interventions with which to support, for example, a woman trying to conceive at any given moment, from fine-tuning her menstrual cycle to possibly providing acupuncture during an IVF procedure, but also taking her age, past reproductive experiences, work environment, personal and social life, family history, astrological chart, diet and lifestyle, signs of momentary alignment or misalignment with her external environment, and other factors into consideration. In a case like this, how can the simple statement "Water is Yīn; Fire is Yáng" enrich a physician's understanding of the interaction of the Heart and Kidney and the interconnected upward-downward movement in the innermost wheel of physiology that makes human life possible? And how might it increase the physician's understanding in a clinical encounter to meditate on the trigrams *kǎn* ☵ and *lí* ☲, whose inherent stability comes perhaps from the fact that they both contain their opposite in the Yīn-Yáng complementarity of their lines? As the commentary points out, "The Kidney is Water, and the creation of Qì inside Water is precisely True Fire; the Heart is Fire, and the creation of fluids inside Fire is precisely True Water." Similarly, the text below discusses Flavor and Qì in medicinal substances as Yīn and Yáng respectively, but then emphasizes the need to differentiate further between Yīn and Yáng aspects within each of them. For just one far-fetched example that might challenge the intuitive knowing of most of us, how might an understanding of solar and lunar cycles, and the effect of these cycles on life on earth, on the alternating seasons and days and nights, and on the flow of water in ebbs and tides contribute to the way we look at physiological functions and pathological actions of the Heart and Kidney?

The significance of the interaction between Essence and Qì on the physician's understanding of the Heart-Kidney axis might be a bit more obvious to the contemporary practitioner of Chinese medicine. Nevertheless, in an agricultural society without modern refrigeration and transportation, the effects of the moon and sun on crops and livestock through the circulation of fluids and action of heat on the natural environment were just as helpful for grasping the polysemic significance of Yīn and Yáng. The frequent references in *Sù Wèn* Chapter 5 to climate, natural processes, and agricultural knowledge are a dimension of this text, and thus a source of insight, that we modern humans may not be able to fully grasp, given how far our technology-dependent lifestyle has removed us from a life within nature.

One last aspect of the above quote from the *Lèi Jīng* is worth pointing out: In contrast to a current trend in Chinese medicine of integrating theories and practices from traditional Chinese alchemy, or religion, into medicine, Zhāng Jièbīn differentiates clearly between the world of *dān* 丹, in the narrowest sense meaning "cinnabar" but by extension also "elixir" and hence here "alchemy" or the practitioner thereof, and *yī* 醫 (medicine). It might surprise modern readers that the pair Essence and Qì is thus specifically positioned outside the purview of medicine. But the *Lèi Jīng* is not the only text to separate alchemical and medical knowledge in this way while at the same time emphasizing the need for specialists in both fields to know the territory of the other. To cite just one prominent example, Chip Chace and Miki Shima have shown that Lǐ Shízhēn 李時珍, the late sixteenth century author of the *Běncǎo Gāng Mù* 《本草綱目》, also differentiated carefully between these two spheres in his *Qí Jīng Bā Mài Kǎo* 《奇經八脈考》 (Investigation of the Eight Extraordinary Channels). In this book, Lǐ explicitly states the significance of the extraordinary vessels not only for the physician but also for what Shima and Chace call the "Daoist adept." For example, he emphasizes the need for both sides to be well-informed in his preface: "If physicians are not aware [of such theories of the extraordinary channels], they will remain in the dark as to the cause of disease. If [aspiring] transcendents are not aware [of the more comprehensive theories of the extraordinary channels], it will be difficult for them to tame the furnace and the cauldron."[4] It may behoove us as modern readers to learn something from this attitude of open-minded interest paired with mutual respect for and recognition of the technical expertise and arduous training necessary to become proficient at one or the other of these two specialties, instead of picking and choosing random aspects from one field to incorporate into one's practice of the other.

* * *

Commentary by Zhāng Jièbīn 張介賓

氣無形而升，故為陽。味有質而降，故為陰。此以藥食氣味言也。

Qì is without Form and bears upward, hence it constitutes Yáng. Flavor has substance and downbears, hence it constitutes Yīn. This line is speaking about [Yīn and Yáng] in terms of the Qì and Flavor in medicinals and food.

* * *

The second part of this line associates Qì with Yáng and Flavor with Yīn. This statement directs our gaze to one of the ways in which the human body interacts most directly with its external environment, namely by ingesting foods and medicinal substances. To understand the meaning of Qì and Flavor here, we need to turn to early materia medica literature, specifically the *Shén Nóng Běncǎo Jīng* 《神農本草經》 (Divine Farmer's Classic of Materia Medica).

[4] Charles Chace and Miki Shima, *An Exposition on the Eight Extraordinary Vessels*, 96.

Quotation from the Preface of the Shén Nóng Běncǎo Jīng 神農本草經

藥有酸、鹹、甘、苦、辛五味；又有寒、熱、溫、涼四氣。

Medicinals have the Five Flavors: sour, salty, sweet, bitter, and acrid. They furthermore have the Four Qì: cold, hot, warm, and cool.

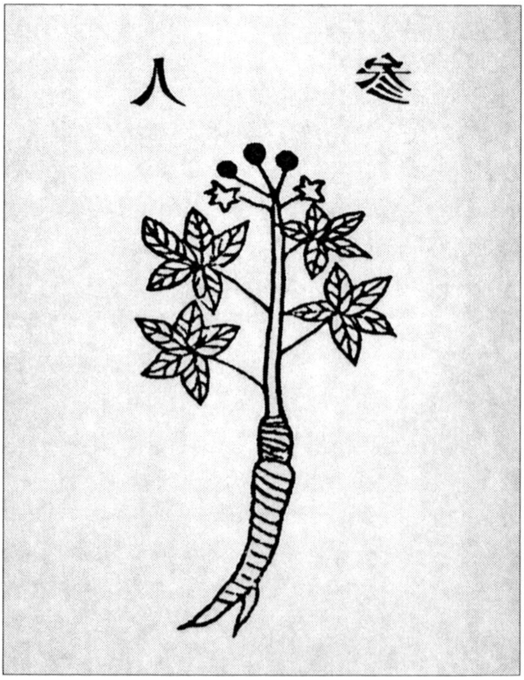

Ginseng

* * *

Quotation from the Shén Nóng Běncǎo Jīng 神農本草經

人參
一名人銜，一名鬼蓋。
味甘，微寒，無毒。

主補五臟，安精神，定魂魄，止驚悸，除邪氣，
明目，開心益智。久服輕身，延年。生山谷。

Rénshēn (root of panax ginseng)
Alternate names: rénxián (human snaffle), guǐgài (ghost cover)
Sweet flavor, slightly cold, non-toxic

Indicated for supplementing the Five Zàng Organs, calming the essence spirit/s and settling the hún and pò souls, stopping fright palpitations, expelling evil qì, brightening the eyes, and opening up the heart and boosting wisdom. Consumed over a long time, it lightens the body and extends the years. Grows in mountain valleys.

* * *

While the dating of the Preface is not without controversy and we therefore cannot accept it as a Hàn dynasty text, the interpretation of Flavor and Qì given there is supported by the structure of the individual entries in the book (consistently classifying each medicinal in one of the Five Flavors and then as cold, warm, slightly cold, slightly warm, or neutral). In addition, the paired usage of the two terms Qì and Flavor with the specific technical meaning of describing the actions and effects of medicinals and foods on the human body is confirmed in other early texts that discuss materia medica or dietetica. The concrete meaning of the Five Flavors and their association already in the *Nèijīng* corpus with the Five *Zàng* Organs (sour—Liver, salty—Kidney, sweet—Spleen/Stomach, bitter—Heart, and acrid—Lung) is universally accepted and consistent. A bit more difficult is the specific meaning of Qì in this brief line. Given its pairing with Flavor here, most commentators interpret it along the lines of standard contemporary materia medica literature as referring to the four thermodynamic qualities mentioned in the Preface to the *Shén Nóng Běncǎo Jīng*: cold, hot, warm, and cool. Nevertheless, this may be a case of reading a later interpretation backwards into an earlier text. For an alternate meaning of Qì in descriptions of the effect of food and medicinal substances, we may consult Sūn Sīmiǎo's 孫思邈 introductory essay to his volume on "Dietary Therapy" (*shí zhì* 食治) in his *Bèi Jí Qiān Jīn Yào Fāng* 備急千金要方 (Essential Formulas Worth a Thousand in Gold to Prepare for Emergencies). Here, Qì refers not to the thermodynamic quality but rather to the nature of a substance, as associated with a certain flavor.

* * *

Quotation from the Bèi Jí Qiān Jīn Yào Fāng[5]

黃帝曰：五味入於口，各有所走，各有所病。酸走筋，多食酸令人癃，不知何以然

少俞曰：酸入胃也，其氣澀以收也。…

The Yellow Emperor said: "Upon entering the mouth, the Five Flavors each have specific locations that they run into and specific diseases that they are associated with. Sourness runs into the sinews, and eating too many sour foods causes a person to suffer from dribbling urinary block. I don't know, what is the reason for this?"

Shào Yú replied: "As for sourness entering the stomach, its Qì is unsmooth and thereby inward-drawing….

* * *

[5] Sūn Sīmiǎo 孫思邈 *Bèi Jí Qiān Jīn Yào Fāng* 《備急千金要方》 (Essential Formulas Worth a Thousand in Gold to Prepare for Emergencies), Volume 26 on *shí zhì* 食治 (Dietary Therapy).

WHILE THE QÌ ASSOCIATED IN THIS TEXT WITH SOURNESS IS described as "unsmooth" (*sè* 澀), the Qì of saltiness is described only as "running into the Middle *Jiāo* and pouring into the various vessels." The Qì of acridity is described as "running into the Upper *Jiāo*, which receives all the Qì and provides for all the Yáng. The Qì of ginger and alliums fumigates provisioning and defense.... Acridity moves together with Qì, and acridity therefore enters the stomach and moves the Qì, and exits together with the Qì..." The Qì of bitterness and of sweetness, lastly, is described as parched and weak, respectively. Thus we see that, at least for Sūn Sīmiǎo or the author of the text he cited, Qì did not refer to temperature but to an aspect of the way in which an ingested substance interacted with the human body. We may never be able to fully reconstruct what the authors of *Sù Wèn* Chapter 5 intended to refer to with the polysemous term Qì in this particular context. Given its pairing with Yáng though, and its opposition to Flavor and Yīn, we might guess that it could be associated with smell, being light, invisible, vaporous, and rising and perceived through the nose, as opposed to the heavy, tangible, dense, descending taste of food that is perceived through the mouth. The following line will shed additional light on this interaction between Qì and Flavor. Further support against reading Qì here as referring to the thermodynamic quality is provided by is provided in Section Three below, where Qì and Flavor are described in these terms: "Acridity and sweetness effuse and disperse, and are Yáng; sourness and bitterness gush up and drain down, and are Yīn," without mentioning temperature.

味歸形，形歸氣，氣歸精，精歸化。精食氣，
形食味。化生精，氣生形。味傷形，氣傷精。
精化為氣，氣傷於味。

Wèi guī xíng, xíng guī qì,
qì guī jīng, jīng guī huà.
Jīng shí qì, xíng shí wèi.
Huà shēng jīng, qì shēng xíng.
Wèi shāng xíng, qì shāng jīng.
Jīng huà wéi qì, qì shāng yú wèi.

Flavor homes to the Form,
the Form homes to Qì;
Qì homes to Essence;
and Essence homes to
Generative Transformation.
Essence feeds on Qì;
the Form feeds on Flavor.
Generative Transformation
engenders Essence;
Qì engenders the Form.
Flavor injures the Form;
Qì injures Essence.
Essence Transforms into Qì;
Qì is injured by Flavor.

Commentary by Zhāng Zhìcōng 張志聰

陰為味，陰成形。地食人以五味，以養此形，故味歸形。陽化氣，諸陽之氣通會於皮膚肌腠之間，以生此形，故形歸氣。陽氣生於陰精，故氣歸於精。水穀之精氣，以化生此精，故精歸於化也。

水穀之精氣，以生此精，精食氣也。五味入胃，以養此形，形食味也。水穀之精氣，以化生此精。諸陽之神氣，以生養此形。蓋天食人以五氣，地食人以五味，氣味化生此精氣，以生養此形也。

夫形食味，精食氣。如飲食之氣味太過，則反傷其精形矣。

精為元氣之本，氣乃精之化也。形食味而味歸形。味傷形則及於氣矣。此節論飲食之陰陽氣味，以生精氣之陰陽而養此形。

Yīn is Flavor, and Yīn completes the Form. Earth feeds humans by means of the Five Flavors, thereby nurturing this Form. Hence "Flavor homes to the Form." Yáng Generatively Transforms Qì, and the Qì of all Yáng penetrates to and gathers in the area of the texture lines of the skin and flesh layers, thereby engendering this Form. Hence "the Form homes to Qì." Yáng Qì is engendered by Yīn Essence, hence "Qì homes to Essence." The Essence Qì of Water and Grain (i.e., all food and drink) is the substance that produces this Essence through Transformation, hence "Essence homes to Generative Transformation."

Because this Essence is engendered from Essence Qì of Water and grain, "Essence feeds on Qì." Because the Five Flavors enter the Stomach and thereby nurture this Form, "the Form feeds on Flavor." Through Generative Transformation, the Essence Qì of Water and grain engenders this Essence; and the Spirit Qì of all Yáng through engendering nurtures this Form. Now, Heaven feeds humans by means of the Five Qì, and Earth feeds humans by means of the Five Flavors. This is the way in which Qì and Flavor transform and engender this Essence and Qì, thereby engendering and nurturing this Form.

Now, the Form feeds on Flavor, and Essence feeds on Qì. If the Qì and Flavor of food and drink are excessive, however, they will injure this Essence and Form instead!

Because Essence is the foundation of Source Qì, Qì is thus engendered through the Transformation of Essence. The Form feeds on Flavor, and Flavor homes to the Form. When Flavor injures the Form, this will then affect the Qì.

This section [of the text] discusses the Yīn and Yáng and Qì and Flavor of food and drink, and how they engender the Yīn and Yáng aspects of Essence and Qì and nurture this Form.

* * *

Using a Yīn-Yáng perspective, this section explores the interactions of the four bodily constituents Flavor (*wèi* 味), Form (*xíng* 形), Qì (氣), and Essence (*jīng* 精), as they transform into and act on each other in a multidirectional cycle of "homing to" (*guī* 歸), "feeding on" (*shí* 食), "engendering" (*shēng* 生), and "injuring" (*shāng* 傷) each other. Here the term *guī* 歸, which I have again translated a bit awkwardly as "to home to" (see page 68), is used in the meaning of being associated with something. Please note that it is employed with a different connotation in the context of contemporary materia medica literature to refer to the specific channel that a substance has an affinity for, in the compound *guī jīng* 歸經 "to home to the channel."

The biggest disagreement among commentators on this passage involves the character *shí* 食, which in the second tone, as it is pronounced most often, means "to eat," or, as I have translated it, "to feed on." In the fourth tone, however, as *shì*, the character is used in the transitive, active sense, as "to cause somebody to eat", or in other words, "to feed." Either meaning is grammatically possible here, and I have chosen "feed" over the common "eat" to remind the reader of this polysemy. As so often in literary Chinese, the character merely conveys the notion of "food," but does not specify the direction of the action from subject to object, in other words, whether it is a matter of giving or receiving food. To make matters worse, one's interpretation must be decided on a phrase-by-phrase basis and does not need to be consistent from one phrase to the next. My own interpretation here is that it means something like "to receive nourishment from," or "be sustained by" throughout this passage, but this is up for debate.

* * *

Commentary by Zhāng Jièbīn 張介賓

五味生精血以成形，故味歸於形。
形之存亡，由氣之聚散，故形歸於氣。.

The Five Flavors engender Essence and Blood and thereby complete the Form. Hence Flavor homes to the Form. The survival or perishing of the Form depends on the gathering or dispersal of Qì, hence the Form homes to Qì.

* * *

The author of this text, Zhāng Jièbīn, further explains that *shí* 食 here has the meaning of "the child feeding on the mother's breastmilk" (子食母乳). Flavor affects and nourishes the physical body (hence the "Form"). Essence consumes or "feeds on" Qì in the same way that the Form consumes or "feeds on" Flavor. Qì produces the physical body in the sense that the Qì of food effects humans. At the same time, Flavor nourishes the Form but can also injure it in pathological cases. On another level, Qì usually comes from but also produces Essence, but can also be injured by it, while Essence is able to transform into Qì.

This interaction takes place both on an external plane and internally: Externally, the physician (or cook) must pay attention to the Flavor and Qì of food and medicinals because they produce Qì and Essence. As a result, over-consuming any one substance can cause damage. Internally, Essence produces Qì, and we therefore must preserve Essence and treasure Qì. It is important to keep in mind in reading this passage that the use of "Flavor" and "Qì" here differs in subtle ways from their understanding in later medicinal therapy.

Section Three

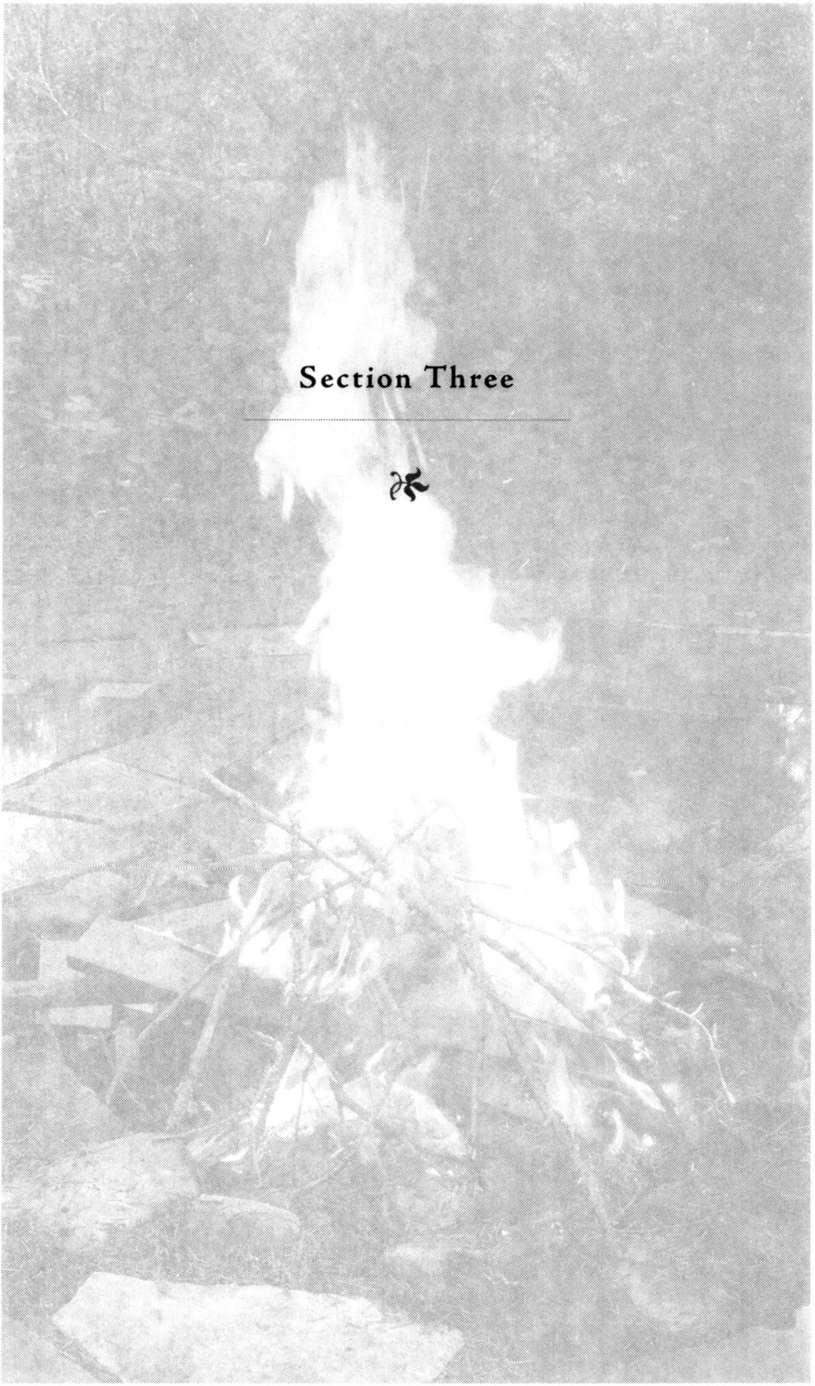

陰味出下竅，陽氣出上竅。
味濃者為陰，薄為陰之陽。氣濃者為陽，薄為陽之陰。
味濃則泄，薄則通。氣薄則發泄，濃則發熱。

Yīn wèi chū xià qiào,
yáng qì chū shàng qiào.

Wèi nóng zhě wéi yīn,
bó wéi yīn zhī yáng.
Qì nóng zhě wéi yáng,
bó wéi yáng zhī yīn.

Wèi nóng zé xiè, bó zé tōng.
Qì bó zé fā xiè, nóng zé fā rè.

Yīn Flavor exits from
the lower apertures;
Yáng Qì exits from
the upper apertures.

Flavor when concentrated, is Yīn but,
when diluted, is the Yáng aspect of Yīn.
Qì, when concentrated, is Yáng but,
when diluted, is the Yīn aspect of Yáng.

Flavor, when concentrated,
results in drainage but,
when diluted, in open passage.
Qì when diluted, results in
drainage through the surface but,
when concentrated, in heat effusion.

Commentary by Zhāng Jièbīn 張介賓

此言氣味之陰陽，而陰陽之中，複各有陰陽也。味為陰矣，而濃者為純陰，薄者為陰中之陽；氣為陽矣，而濃者為純陽，薄者為陽中之陰。。。。陰味下行，故味濃者能泄於下，薄者能通利；陽氣上行，故氣薄者能泄於表，濃者能發熱也。

This passage discusses the Yīn and Yáng of Qì and Flavor, and there is in turn a Yīn and a Yáng [aspect] within each of them. Thus, Flavor is Yīn, and concentrated Flavor is pure Yīn, while diluted Flavor is the Yáng aspect of Yīn; Qì is Yáng, and in its concentrated form is pure Yáng and in its diluted form Yīn within Yáng. Yīn Flavor moves downward, and concentrated Flavor therefore has the effect of causing drainage from the lower body, while diluted Flavor is able to promote open passage. Yáng Qì naturally moves upward and, when diluted, is able to drain outward through the exterior, while it is able to effuse heat when concentrated.

THE SOLID *ZÀNG* ORGANS 臟 ("VISCERA" IN WISEMAN TERMINOLOGY) are associated with the process of entering (*rù* 入) and with storing substances, while the hollow *Fǔ* Organs 腑 ("bowels" in Wiseman terminology) are associated with exiting (*chū* 出), i.e., with the elimination of substances by turning ingested food and liquids into urine and feces. Similarly, the *Zàng* Organs are correlated with an ascending movement (*shēng* 升), with sending things up and out to clear the upper orifices and sense organs, and the *Fǔ* Organs with a descending movement (*jiàng* 降) and with elimination through the lower orifices. Keeping this flow smooth and open in both directions, as expressed by the character *tōng* 通 ("open passage"), is the hallmark of a healthy Qì dynamic, represented by the character *shùn* 順 (movement in the right direction or with the natural flow), as opposed to *nì* 逆, which means movement against the proper course or "counterflow" in Wiseman terminology.

In clinical terms, the body's Qì dynamic consists of an outer wheel, where Liver Qì ascends while Lung Qì descends; and an inner wheel, where Kidney Qì ascends, while Heart Qì descends. The Spleen and Stomach, located squarely in the center, provide the anchor that sustains this movement in both directions by supplying the other four organs with nourishment.

In any discussion of movement in the body, we need to be aware that the movement of ascending and descending in terms of organ function is relative. As such, Liver-Wood also moves horizontally to support Earth in the Spleen and Stomach, to aid digestion, and also moves downward to help the Kidney's function of excreting urine. Similarly, all the *Fǔ* Organs are associated with a downward movement of Qì, but the small intestine, for example, after receiving food

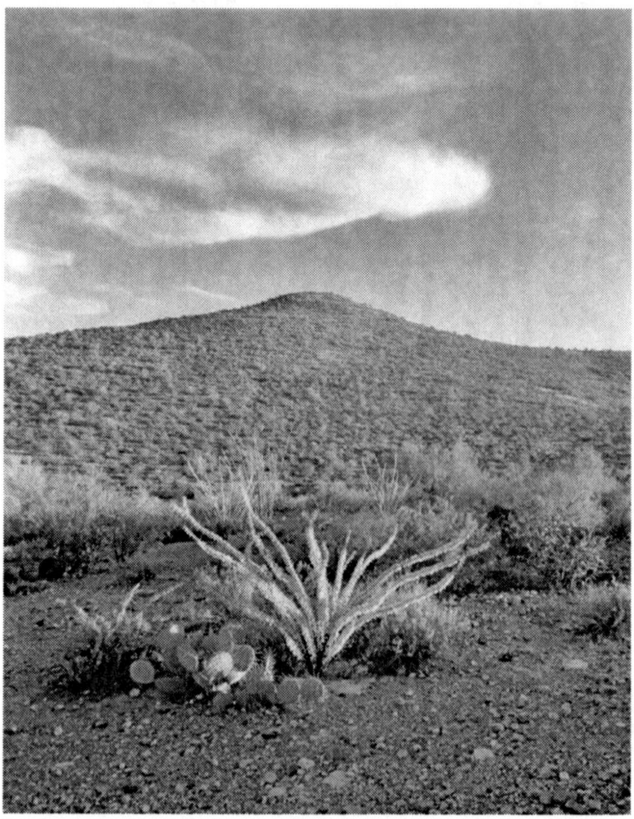

from the Stomach, makes the clear rise up to the Lung. And while the bladder processes the turbid fluids downward, it is also involved in recycling the clear up to the Lung by means of the Kidney. We should thus use this information on pathological and physiological movement up and down as a clinical guideline. The physiological flow of Liver Qì upward, if stagnant, can quickly escalate into pathological uprising, resulting in anger, heat, bulging eyes, and a hot face, necessitating sometimes drastic intervention to anchor Liver Qì. Similarly, the intestines need to be purged regularly in the downward flow of the Qì dynamic that is associated with the *Fǔ* Organs. If the large intestine is blocked, this normal function is disabled and might need to be restored with substances like dàhuáng 大黄.

Some commentators read the actions described in the last paragraph of this passage of the *Great Treatise* as pathologies, others as healthy physiology or as the intended effects of medicinal substances. Especially the last expression, *fā rè* 發熱 "effuse as heat," can be interpret as "fever" or as promoting warmth and the healthy release of heat through the surface by assisting Yáng. Similar, *xiè* 泄 ("drainage") can be read as physiological drainage or, in the eyes of most commentators, as pathological leakage, or in other words, diarrhea. Thus, substances with a thick, concentrated Flavor are likely to cause diarrhea, while substances with thin, diluted Flavor promote a healthy free flow; substances with diluted Qì tend to make us sweat, while substances with concentrated Qì make us hot. In clinic, Flavor induces a downward movement while Qì has an upbearing effect. Further differentiated, thick concentrated Flavor (like *dàhuáng* 大黄) causes purging, while weaker Flavor has an opening, coursing 通 effect (like *zéxiè* 澤瀉 or *mùtōng* 木通). The strong concentrated Qì of substances like *fùzi* 附子 brings heat to the surface 發熱, while the gentle Qì of substances like *máhuáng* 麻黃 is ideal for promoting sweating 發泄.

壯火之氣衰；少火之氣壯。壯火食氣，氣食少火。
壯火散氣；少火生氣。

Zhuàng huǒ zhī qì shuāi;
shào huǒ zhī qì zhuàng.
Zhuàng huǒ shí qì;
qì shí shào huǒ.
Zhuàng huǒ sàn qì;
shào huǒ shēng qì.

The Qì of Strong Fire weakens;
the Qì of Lesser Fire strengthens.
Strong Fire feeds on Qì;
Qì feeds on Lesser Fire.
Strong Fire scatters Qì;
Lesser Fire generates Qì.

* * *

Commentary by Gāo Shìzōng 高士宗

壯火，亢盛之火，即相火也。少火，和緩之火，即君火也。亢盛之壯火宜衰，和緩之少火宜壯。夫壯火何以宜衰？以壯火食氣故也。少火何以宜壯？以氣食少火故也。所謂壯火食氣，實壯火散氣也，所謂氣食少火，實少火生氣也。

Strong Fire is Fire that is hyperactive and exuberant, which refers to Ministerial Fire (xiànghuǒ). Lesser Fire is Fire that is warm and gentle, which refers to Sovereign Fire (jūnhuǒ). Hyperactive and exuberant Strong Fire should be weakened, and warm and gentle Lesser Fire should be strengthened. Why is it that Strong Fire should be weakened? Because Strong Fire feeds on Qì. Why is it that Lesser Fire should be strengthened? Because Qì consumes Lesser Fire. The expression "Strong Fire feeds on Qì" in actuality means that Strong Fire scatters Qì, while the expression "Qì feeds on Lesser Fire" in actuality means that Lesser Fire engenders Qì.

* * *

Before delving into a clinical discussion, it is necessary to comment on two terminological issues. The first note concerns the character *shí/shì* 食, which we have already encountered in Section Two, beginning with page 80. As in that line, I also read it here in the second tone, as "to eat" or "to feed on," instead of in the fourth tone as "to feed." In the first phrase, we can interpret this "feeding on" in the sense that Strong Fire consumes Qì and hence weakens the body as the result of hyperactive Yáng, while "feeding on" in the second phrase means that Qì receives sustenance from Lesser Fire. This line is often explained as referring to medicinal substances, giving wūtóu 烏頭 and fùzǐ 附子 as examples for hot substances that represent "Strong Fire" and consume Qì if the person's own Qì is not strong enough to meet them and "overcome" the Qì of the substance. As a result, they can end up weakening the person in the end. In contrast, rénshēn 人參 is cited as an example for a warm substance of "Lesser Fire" that nourishes Qì by warming it bit by bit.

* * *

Commentary by Wáng Bīng 王冰

氣生壯火，故云壯火食氣。少火滋氣，故云氣食少火。
以壯火食氣，故氣得壯火則耗散。以少火益氣，
故氣得少火則生長。人之陽氣壯少亦然。

Because Qì engenders Strong Fire, the text says that "Strong Fire feeds on Qì." Because Lesser Fire fertilizes Qì, the text says that "Qì feeds on Lesser Fire." Due to the fact that Strong Fire feeds on Qì, Qì dissipates when exposed to Strong Fire. Due to the fact that Lesser Fire boosts Qì, Qì grows when exposed to Lesser Fire. The state of Strong and Lesser Yáng Qì in humans is also like this.

* * *

I FOLLOW MOST COMMENTATORS IN TRANSLATING THE TWO CHARACTERS *zhuàng* 壯 and *shào* 少 in the most common meaning of these terms as "strong" and "lesser." Nevertheless, we may also want to consider that this pair of terms is often used in the sense of "adult," i.e., referring people or things in their prime, most highly developed state, and "young," referring to people or things in an incipient state of development respectively.

Turning now to the clinical significance of this line, it might be directed at the ancient precursors of the "School of Supporting Yáng" (*fú yáng pài* 扶養派) or "Fire Spirit School" (*huǒ shén pài* 火神派), by warning against the excessive use of strong Yáng-supporting medicinals and treatments. Hot fiery herbs like *fùzi* 附子, *gānjiāng* 乾薑, or *guìzhī* 桂枝 may be used temporarily to boost Yáng Qì, but their use over time can end up working counterproductively by scattering Qì.

This warning is particularly interesting in light of the living conditions at the time when this chapter was composed. We can imagine the added importance and popularity of strong Yáng-supporting medicinals at a time when the center of Chinese culture was located in the traditional heartland of northern China and people were living in primitive shelters without centralized heat. Brutal exposure to cold environments, especially when paired with inadequate access to rich warm foods, must have weakened the population in harsh winters, as is expressed in the famous preface to the *Shāng Hán Lùn*. Here the author Zhāng Zhòngjǐng laments losing two thirds of his relatives from the effects of Cold Damage in his own clan alone:

* * *

Quotation from the Preface to the Shāng Hán Lùn 傷寒論

余宗族素多，向余二百，建安紀年以來，猶未十稔，其死亡者，三分有二，傷寒十居其七。感往昔之淪喪，傷橫夭之莫救，乃勤求古訓，博采眾方。

My ancestral clan has always been numerous, with more than two hundred members in the past. But since the first year of Jiàn'ān (i.e., 196 CE), in less than ten years, the proportion of those who have perished has been two out of three, with Cold Damage claiming seven out of ten of these. Deeply affected by this ruinous loss in my past and by the failure to rescue them from injury and premature death, I have diligently sought out the ancient instructions and collected a great number of methods far and wide.

* * *

Especially in the cold winters of northern China, it is quite likely that harsh heating substances were popular remedies because of their immediate effect on bodies suffering from exposure to cold. The warning expressed in the present line might thus offer us with a rare insight into actual clinical practice in early China, reflecting an awareness, at least among higher-level medical practitioners, that excessively hot substances and prescriptions could have a detrimental effect on people whose Qì was not strong enough to handle it.

The sort of medicinal treatment referred to in the present line as "Strong Fire" may be extremely effective in patients with severe Yáng deficiency, but is inappropriate for Yīn deficiency and is moreover not sustainable over a long time. Thus, substances with weak Fire make Qì strong, while those with Strong Fire make Qì weak, or in other words, Qì is strengthened by weak Fire but is consumed by Strong Fire. As a common theme in classical medical literature, we see how this passage emphasizes the need to apply strong treatments only with care and in moderation.

In terms of treatment approaches, the "Cold Cooling School" (*Hán Liáng Pài* 寒涼派) from the Jīn-Yuán period was quite influential in emphasizing the danger of pathological Fire. Reflecting this concern in an earlier text, nine out of the famous Nineteen Lines from *Sù Wèn* Chapter 74, which is generally held to be a Táng dynasty insertion to the *Nèi Jīng*, relate to Fire as a pathology that has to be addressed with cooling methods and cold herbs. Controlling excessive Fire also became an important concern of "Warm Disease" (*Wēn Bìng* 溫病) treatments. At the same time, however, it is also important to support Lesser Fire and build up Yīn, as promoted by Zhū Dānxī 朱丹溪 (1281–1358) and his followers in the *Enriching Yīn School* (*Zī Yīn Pài* 滋陰派). To bring down excessive and upflaring Ministerial Fire that results from Yīn deficiency, we must boost Yīn with herbs like zhīmǔ 知母 and huángbǎi 黄柏 and formulas like Sì Wù Tāng 四物湯.

To conclude this discussion, I would like to cite Zhāng Jièbīn's commentary. It reminds us that this passage can be read not just in the context of materia medica and dietetica, but also as a general comment on the benefits and dangers of Fire as a force in the human body and in Heaven and Earth.

* * *

Commentary by Zhāng Jièbīn 張介賓

火，天地之陽氣也。天非此火，不能生物；人非此火，不能有生。故萬物之生，皆由陽氣。但陽和之火則生物，亢烈之火反害物，故火太過則氣反衰，火和平則氣乃壯。

Fire is the Yáng Qì of Heaven and Earth. Heaven, if it were not for this Fire, would be unable to engender things. Humanity, if it were not for this fire, would not be able to have life. As such, the life of the Myriad Things all depends on Yáng Qì. Nevertheless, while a harmonious Yáng Fire results in engendering things, an overly fierce Fire has the opposite effect of harming things. As such, when Fire is excessive, Qì is on the contrary weakened, but when Fire is harmonious and balanced, Qì is indeed strengthened by it.

* * *

* * *

Commentary by Z'ev Rosenberg

The comments by Zhū Dānxī 朱丹溪 and Liú Wánsù 劉完素 are in contrast to the position of Zhèng Qīn'ān 鄭欽安 and physicians of the "Fire Spirit School" (*Huǒ Shén Pài* 火神派). My understanding of the importance of Yáng Qì is taken from *Sù Wèn* Chapter 3: "Yáng Qì [in the human body] is like the sun in the sky. ….As such, the Yáng Qì throughout the course of the day is in charge of the outside: At daybreak, the person's Qì is engendered; in the middle of the day, Yáng Qì is at its height; and when the sun is in the west, the Yáng Qì has become vacuous and the gates of Qì are closed up (unpublished translation by Sabine Wilms).

The Yáng Qì is compared to the sun. As such, it dominates the Yīn and is necessary for mobilizing Yīn Qì. For example, Shèn Qì Wán 腎氣丸 (Kidney Qì Pill) contains ròuguì 肉桂 (according to Eric Brand, the bark was used, but called guìzhī 桂枝 in ancient texts) and *fùzǐ* 附子. The example of Liù Wèi Dìhuáng Wán 六味地黄丸 (Six Ingredient Dìhuáng Pill), which was adapted by Qián Yǐ 錢乙 as a pediatric formula for small children who generally have strong Yáng Qì and require Yīn supplementation, is an exception. The Ministerial Fire (*xiàng huǒ* 相火), which circulates through the body via the Shàoyáng (Sānjiāo and Gallbladder) and Juéyīn (Blood) layers, regulates the body's vital heat. Treatment strategies should include either warming

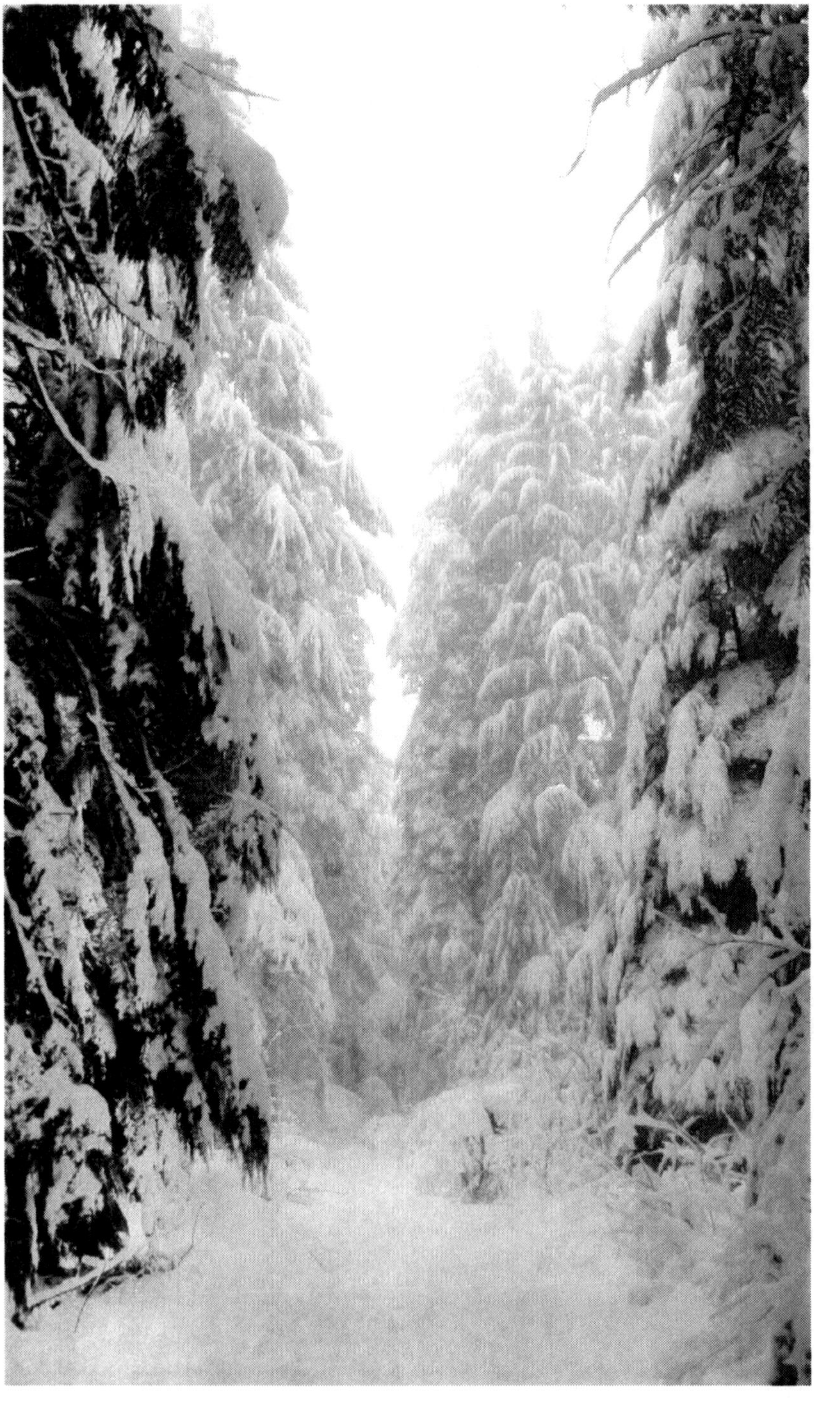

the Yáng (fùzǐ, ròuguì, gānjiāng 乾薑), regulating the Shàoyáng (cháihú 柴胡 formulas), draining the Yángmíng (shígāo 石膏/Bái Hǔ 白虎 formulas or dàhuáng 大黄/Chéng Qì 承氣 formulas), or harmonizing *yíng* provisioning and *wèi* defense (Guìzhī Tāng formulas), depending on depth of pathology, pulse, and symptom pattern. But draining Fire is often like bloodletting, and there is a potential risk that too much Heat is allowed to escape. Zhū Dānxī's ideas on Yīn Vacuity and Fire were not in agreement with a large majority of historical Chinese physicians, and even in his case, only a few of his formulas are strong Yīn supplements or Fire drainers. In contrast, few of Liú Wánsù's 劉完素 formulas are still used today—they are too cold and draining! True Fire evils are rare in Western patients, who are subject to biomedical treatment with anti-inflammatories, steroids, and antibiotics cooling off the body before we Chinese medicine practitioners even treat them, and requiring treatment to protect and repair the Yáng Qì. Other drugs, such as methotrexate, which is used to treat Stills Disease, can create angry red skin rashes, rapid pulses, and bright red tongues, indicative of Fire evils and a need for the patient to be cooled and for Yīn to be rescued. In such cases, we can choose formulas such as Liù Wèi Dìhuáng Wán in combination with Guìzhī Fúlíng Wán 桂枝茯苓丸.

* * *

氣味，辛甘發散為陽，酸苦湧泄為陰。

Qì wèi, xīn gān fā sàn wéi yáng,
suān kǔ yǒng xiè wéi yīn.

In terms of Qì and Flavor,
acridity and sweetness
effuse and disperse,
and are Yáng;
sourness and bitterness
gush up and drain down,
and are Yīn.

Commentary by Zhāng Zhìcōng 張志聰

言氣味固分陰陽，而味中複有陰陽之別。辛走氣而性散。甘乃中央之味，而能灌溉四旁。故辛甘主發散為陽也。苦主泄下，而又炎上作苦。酸主收降，而又屬春生之木味。皆能上湧而下泄。故酸苦湧泄為陰也。

This [line] is saying that Qì and Flavor certainly divide into Yīn and Yáng. And that within Flavor there again is a differentiation of Yīn and Yáng. Acridity makes the Qì run and is dispersing by its nature. Sweetness is indeed the Flavor of the true center and is able to irrigate all four sides. For this reason, acridity and sweetness govern effusing and dispersing and constitute Yáng. Bitterness governs downward drainage, and yet flaming upward is what produces bitterness. Sourness governs drawing in and downbearing, and at the same time is also the Flavor associated with Wood, which sprouts in the spring. They are both able to gush upward and drain downward. For this reason sourness and bitterness [govern] gushing and draining and constitute Yīn.

THIS PASSAGE IN THE *GREAT TREATISE* IS THE EARLIEST INSTANCE IN the received literature of the Five Flavors being categorized in accordance with their Yīn-Yáng action. It describes the effects of Flavor in medicinal substances and foods on the human body: Acridity obviously effuses, or in other words, moves out through the surface and disperses. Sweetness goes to the Stomach and from there relaxes and irrigates the four directions from the center, and is therefore also associated with the expansive upward and outward activity of Yáng. In contrast, sourness is astringent but sometimes causes purging from the lower orifices. Bitterness is descending, as expressed by the common saying "bitterness is able to drain" 苦能泄. For this reason, sourness and bitterness are associated with the contracting, downward, and inward activity of Yīn. To give just one example in the style of the "School of Attacking and Purging" (*gòng xià pài* 攻下派) advocated by

Zhāng Cóngzhèng 張從正 (1156-1228) and his followers, bitterness is able to clear Fire by bringing it down and thereby getting rid of it. Purging, or literally "inducing a downward movement" (*xià* 下), also translated as "precipitation" by Wiseman and Feng, is one of the three treatment methods for aggressively eliminating pathogens, with the other two being promoting sweating (*hàn* 汗) and inducing vomiting (*tù* 吐). The choice of treatment must always depend on the location of the pathogen: When it is in the Upper *Jiāo*, for example, vomiting is indicated. In all three of these approaches, though, we must take care to avoid injury to Stomach Qì.

Section Four

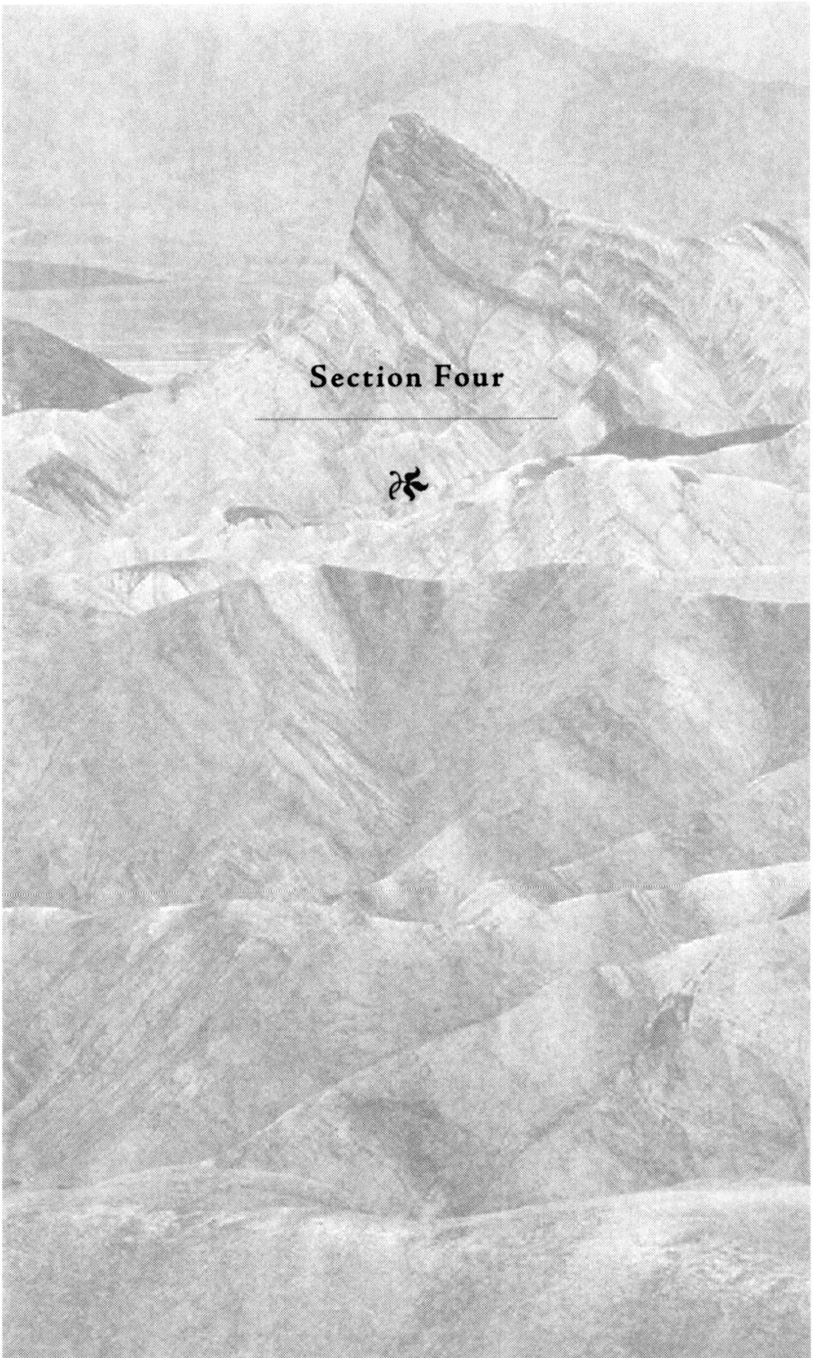

陰勝則陽病，陽勝則陰病。
陽勝則熱，陰勝則寒。
重寒則熱，重熱則寒。

Yīn shèng zé yáng bìng,
yáng shèng zé yīn bìng.

Yáng shèng zé rè,
yīn shèng zé hán.

Chóng/zhòng hán zé rè, chóng/
zhòng rè zé hán.

When Yīn prevails, Yáng falls ill;
when Yáng prevails, Yīn falls ill.

When Yáng prevails, Heat results;
when Yīn prevails, Cold results.

Extreme/double Cold results in Heat;
extreme/double Heat results in Cold.

As much as I try in this book to transmit the literal meaning and structure of the text in the literal translation section with as little personal interpretation as possible, inadvertently I might be contributing to this trend simply by arranging the text in sections that impose an artificial structure. Please keep in mind that the original text lacked punctuation and divisions but was written in one continuous stream. Most scholars and practitioners read the present passage as no longer referring to the Qì and Flavor of medicinals discussed in the previous segment but as starting a new section in the text that discusses the balance of Yīn and Yáng Qì in the human body and in the macrocosm. The following commentary by Gāo Shìzōng is an exception to this dominant interpretation and serves here as a reminder that we must read each line not just as an individual statement but also in the context of its placement in the text as a whole.

* * *

Commentary by Gāo Shìzōng 高士宗

分而言之，氣為陽，味為陰。合而言之，氣不離味，味不離氣，故氣味辛甘，從中達外，主能發散，故為陽。氣味酸苦，從中上下，主能湧泄，故為陰。陰勝則陽病者，酸苦之味太過，則陰勝而陽斯病矣，陽勝則陰病者，辛甘之味太過，則陽勝而陰斯病矣。

Speaking of them in separate terms, Qì is Yáng and Flavor is Yīn. Speaking of them as a unit, Qì never leaves the Flavor, and the Flavor never leaves the Qì. Hence, when Qì and Flavor are acrid or sweet, thrusting outward from the center, they rule the ability to effuse and disperse. Hence they constitute Yáng. When the Qì and Flavor are sour or bitter, moving up and down from the center, they rule the ability to gush up and drain down. Hence they are Yīn. Regarding the statement 'when Yīn prevails, Yáng falls ill,' an excess of sour or bitter Flavor results in Yīn prevailing and Yáng then falling ill, and that is all. Regarding "when Yáng prevails, Yīn falls ill," an excess of acrid or sweet Flavor results in Yáng prevailing and Yīn then falling ill, and that is all.

Of course many scholars argue that the original text was nothing but a compilation of separate segments and therefore can and should be read as such. In addition, for the purpose of adding commentary and discussion to the text in a usable book arrangement, it is necessary to split the source text into sections, as commentators have done at least since Wáng Bīng in the Táng dynasty. As a critical reader, however, it is important to remember that this segmentation of the text does not reflect the original condition but is done by each commentator and editor in accordance with their reading of the text.

* * *

Commentary by Zhāng Jièbīn 張介賓

言陰陽偏勝之為病也。陰陽不和，則有勝有虧，故皆能為病。。。
物極則變也。此即上文寒極生熱、熱極生寒之義。蓋陰陽之氣，
水極則似火，火極則似水，陽盛則隔陰，陰盛則隔陽。故有真寒假熱，
真熱假寒之辨，此而錯認，則死生反掌。。。寒為陰，形亦屬陰，
寒則形消故傷形。熱為陽，氣亦屬陽，熱則氣散故傷氣。。。

What this passage is talking about is the process by which a one-sided prevalence of Yīn or Yáng produces illness. A disharmony between Yīn and Yáng results in prevalence here and depletion there, and hence in all cases in the potential for illness to form… When things reach their extreme point, they change. This is the meaning of the above phrase that 'Extremes of Cold engender Heat; extremes of Heat engender Cold'. In terms of Yīn and Yáng Qì, the extreme form of Water resembles Fire, and the extreme form of Fire resembles Water. When Yáng is exuberant, it impedes Yīn, and when Yīn is exuberant, it impedes Yáng. Hence we have the differentiation of True Cold with False Heat, and True Heat with False Cold. When these disease states are identified incorrectly, life and death can flip as easily as the turn of your hand… Cold is Yīn, and the Form also belongs to Yīn. As a result of Cold, the Form is diminished, thus it injures the Form. Heat is Yáng, and Qì also belongs to Yáng. As the result of Heat, Qì is dispersed, thus it injures Qì.

* * *

Following most commentators, I interpret this entire section as discussing Yīn and Yáng pathologies in various patterns. The first line in this passage addresses how an excess of Yīn or Yáng results in illness, specifically in deficiency, in its complementary or opposite aspect. In the first case, an excess of Yīn, which usually points to a Cold pathogen, has caused illness in Yáng. Dr. Long Rihui here recommends Sì Nì Tāng 四逆湯 as a representative formula to disperse excess Cold, since in these indications the Cold needs to be drained with extremely hot medicinals like fùzǐ, gānjiāng, and guìzhī. At the same time, however, Yáng here has to be supported and built up with Yáng tonics like lùjiǎojiāo 鹿角膠, ròucóngrōng 肉蓯蓉, and yínyánghùo 淫羊藿 to treat the Yáng deficiency. In the opposite case, when the formation of Heat (or in other words, the so-called "prevalence of Yáng") has caused illness in the Yīn aspect, we need to clear Heat and simultaneously nourish Yīn with modifications of formulas like Bái Hǔ Tāng 白虎湯. To engender Yīn fluids, however, we also want to add Yīn tonics like xuánshēn 玄參, màiméndōng 麥門冬, and shēngdìhuáng 生地黄 (from the formula Zēng Yè Tāng 增液湯). Thus it is important, while clearing the excess, to treat the deficiency by means of tonics and to watch out for the dangers of "Strong Fire" 壯火 mentioned in the previous section in reference to medicinal action.

In contrast, Line Two describes situations where a prevalence of Yīn results in Cold and where a prevalence of Yáng results in Heat, but still without affecting the opposite aspect. For such pure excess patterns, it is enough to drain the pathogen with Sì Nì Tāng or Bái Hǔ Tāng alone.

Line Three has been the subject of much discussion, based on one's interpretation of the character 重: It can be read as *zhòng*, meaning "heavy" or "severe," or as *chóng*, meaning "double." Either option is possible here: We can interpret this line as meaning that an extreme root condition of Cold or Heat will turn into or manifest as its opposite, as expressed in the phrases "True Cold with False Heat" 真寒假熱 and "True Heat with False Cold" 真熱假寒. Alternatively, if we read 重 as *chóng* ("double"), it could refer to such circumstances as internal Cold being complicated by external Cold, or of external Cold affecting Yīn aspects of the body, or of additional Cold factors further aggravating the effects of a cold season. Dr. Long Rihui reads 重 as *chóng* in the sense of "double." In his opinion, this line should not be read as referring to a situation of False Cold or False Heat with an underlying pathology of its opposite where, for example, an extreme deep-lying Cold pathology leads to a Heat manifestation when the Cold pushes the Heat to the surface, to be treated with formulas like Tōng Mài Sì Nì Tāng 通脈四逆湯. Instead, Dr. Long interprets this line as describing a situation where a critical pathology of extreme Cold or Heat turns into its opposite. These sorts of life-threatening situations are unlikely to appear in the clinic of contemporary Chinese medicine practitioners, however, since such patients are more likely to go straight to the emergency room of a biomedical hospital.

寒傷形，熱傷氣。氣傷痛，形傷腫。
故先痛而後腫者，氣傷形也；先腫而後痛者，形傷氣也。

Hán shāng xíng; rè shāng qì.
Qì shāng tòng; xíng shāng zhǒng.

Gù xiān tòng ér hòu zhǒng zhě, qì shāng xíng yě; xiān zhǒng ér hòu tòng zhě, xíng shāng qì yě.

Cold injures the Form;
Heat injures Qì.
Qì injury means pain;
injury to the Form means swelling.

For this reason, when there is pain first and then swelling afterwards, this means that Qì has injured the Form; when there is swelling first and then pain afterwards, this means that the Form has injured the Qì.

Commentary by Gāo Shìzōng 高士宗

寒為陰邪，故寒傷形。熱為陽邪，故熱傷氣。氣傷則痛，痛，周身無形之氣也。形傷則腫，腫，周身有形之形也。故先痛而後腫者，先傷氣而後傷形也；先腫而後痛者，先傷形而後傷氣也。

Cold is a Yīn evil and Cold therefore injures the Form. Heat is a Yáng evil and Heat therefore injures the Qì. The reason why Qì injury results in pain is that pain is a case of Form-less Qì all over the body. The reason why Form injury results in swelling is that swelling is a case of Form that has Form all over the body. As such, pain first with swelling afterwards means Qì injury first and injury to the Form afterwards, while swelling first with pain afterwards means injury to the Form first and injury to the Qì afterwards.

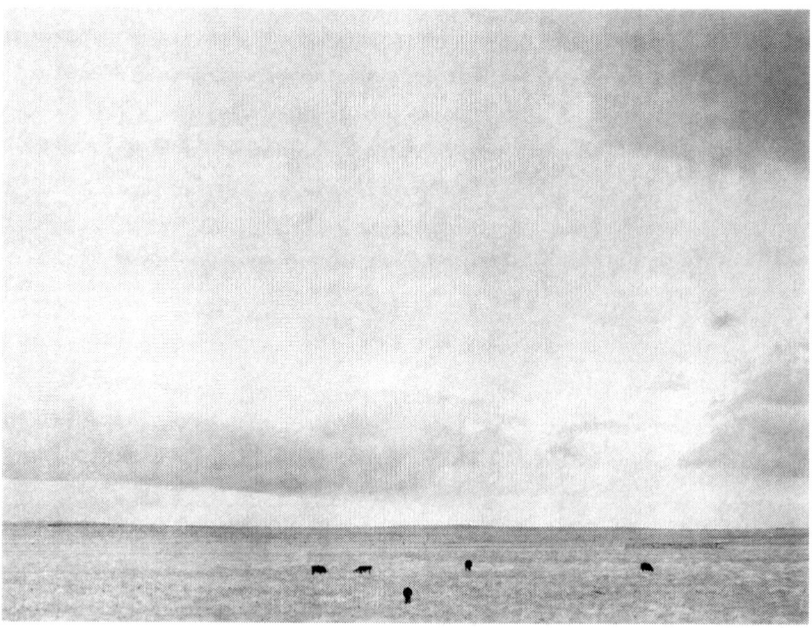

To understand the first half of this passage, Dr. Long suggests that we consider the pathology of Bì 痹 Impediment Syndrome, as expressed in the "Discussion of Bì Impediment" 痹論 in *Sù Wèn* Chapter 43. Here it is related to an invasion of Wind, Cold, or Dampness in the very first explanation of this condition, while a subsequent statement relates pain to the prevalence of Cold in Bì Impediment.

* * *

Quotation from Sù Wèn[1]

風寒濕三氣雜至，合而為痺也。其風氣勝者為行痺，寒氣勝者為痛痺，濕氣勝者為著痺也。…

…痛者，寒氣多也，有寒故痛也。

When a medley of the three Qì of Wind, Cold, and Dampness reaches the body and blends together, it forms Bì Impediment. In this condition, if Wind Qì predominates, the patient develops Moving Bì; if Cold Qì predominates, the patient develops Painful Bì; if Damp Qì predominates, the patient develops Adhesive Bì....

...The presence of pain means a preponderance of Cold Qì, because when there is Cold, this causes pain."

* * *

To explain the second half of each sentence in this line, that "Heat injures Qì" and that "injury to the Form means swelling," Dr. Long emphasizes that physical injury to the body is a prime cause of swelling. In this line, Cold and Heat refer to Cold Damage and Warm Disease (*wēnbìng* 溫病) respectively, or in other words to external pathogens. In the case of Cold Damage, we see signs like neck

[1] *Sù Wèn* 《素問》 Chapter 43, *Bì Lùn* 痹論 (Discussion of Bì Impediment).

pain and blocked channels, while an invasion of Heat, especially in the summer, manifests with sweating and outpouring, which injures the Qì. In such cases, Dr. Long recommends Bái Hǔ Jiā Rénshēn Tāng 白虎加人參湯 to tonify Qì.

In contrast to the relationship between Cold and pain cited elsewhere in the *Sù Wèn*, however, other commentators such as Gāo Shìzōng (quoted above) and Zhāng Jièbīn relate Cold here, as a Yīn evil, to injury to the Form and to swelling, and heat, as a Yáng evil, to injury to Qì and to pain.

* * *

Commentary by Zhāng Jièbīn 張介賓

寒為陰，形亦屬陰，寒則形消故傷形。熱為陽，氣亦屬陽，熱則氣散故傷氣。

氣欲利，故傷之則痛。形有質，故傷之則腫。

Cold is Yīn, and the Form also belongs to Yīn. When there is Cold, the Form is diminished, and thus it injures the Form. Heat is Yáng, and Qì also belongs to Yáng. When there is Heat, the Qì scatters, and thus it injures the Qì.

Qì wants to flow freely, and for this reason injury to it results in pain. The Form has substances, and for this reason injury to it results in swelling.

* * *

Given the preference for strict parallelism in literary Chinese, however, the switched order half-way through the first part of this passage should make us pause and might indicate that it perhaps takes up the issue from a different angle, as Dr. Long's distinction between external pathogens and physical injury suggests. One could even make an argument to change the punctuation in such a way that the second half of the first section in this passage belongs to the second section instead.

Regardless of punctuation, the second half of this passage describes cases where both the Qì and the Form have been injured, resulting in both swelling and pain. Here, it is important to diagnose correctly which one of these two signs appeared first, so that we can differentiate between the "tip" 表 and the "trunk" 本 condition. In such patterns of combined pain and swelling, we should follow the general guideline of treating the "trunk" condition first, in the hope that the resulting "tip" condition will resolve on its own. Since Cold injures the Form and injury to the Form manifests in swelling, a progression of disease from swelling to pain means that we first need to address the Cold condition. Similarly, Heat injures the Qì and Qì injury manifests in pain, so when we see pain preceding swelling, this indicates that Heat is the root cause that needs to be addressed first.

風勝則動，熱勝則腫，燥勝則乾，
寒勝則浮，濕勝則濡瀉。

Fēng shèng zé dòng,
rè shèng zé zhǒng,
zào shèng zé gān,
hán shèng zé fú,
shī shèng zé rú xiè.

Predominance of Wind
results in stirring;
predominance of Heat
results in swelling;
predominance of Parching
results in dryness;
predominance of Cold
results in floating;
predominance of Dampness
results in drenching outpouring.

* * *

Commentary by Zhāng Zhìcōng 張志聰

此以下論天之四時五行，人之五臟五氣，外感六淫，內傷五志，
亦有陰陽寒熱之為病也。風性動搖，故風勝則動。熱氣傷陰，
故熱勝則腫。燥傷津液，故燥勝則干。寒氣傷陽，故神氣乃浮也。
濕淫所勝，則脾土受傷，而為濡瀉之病矣。風熱、天之陽氣也。
寒燥濕、天之陰氣也。乃四時五行之陰陽偏勝而為病也。

This passage discusses the Four Seasons and Five Dynamic Agents in Heaven and the Five Zàng Organs and Five Qì in humans, the externally contracted Six Excesses and the internally injurious Five Emotions, as well as the causation of illness from Yīn and Yáng and Cold and Heat. Because it is the nature of Wind to stir up and shake, a predominance of Wind results in stirring. Because Heat Qì injures Yīn, a predominance of Heat results in swelling. Because Parching injures the fluids, a predominance of Parching results in Dryness. Because Cold Qì injures Yáng, the Shén and Qì then float. When Dampness Evil is predominant, Spleen-Earth sustains injury, and this then produces the disease of drenching outpouring. Wind and Heat are the Yáng Qì of Heaven; Cold, Parching, and Dampness are the Yīn Qì of Heaven. This then is how one-sided predominances of Yīn or Yáng in the Four Seasons or Five Dynamic Agents produce illness.

* * *

This passage emphasizes the need to identify the proper underlying disease cause by differentiating the key signs. Dr. Long offers some clinical observations on each of the five disease causes (*bìng yīn* 病因) listed here, namely Wind, Heat, Parching, Cold, and Dampness: In the medicinal treatment of Wind, it is important to distinguish between external Wind, which must be expelled, and internal Wind, which must be extinguished. In acupuncture, we treat the same Wind points, like Fēngfǔ 風府 (DU-16) or Fēngchí 風池, (GB-20) but paired with Wàiguān 外關 (SJ-5) for external Wind and Nèiguān 內關 (PC-6) for internal Wind conditions. Swelling as the result of Cold refers to skin conditions like furuncles or carbuncles that are marked by redness and swelling. The phrase "Predominance of Parching results in Dryness," refers to patterns where we must nourish Yīn and moisten Dryness with formulas like Wǔ Zhī Yǐn 五汁飲 (consisting of pear, water chestnut, sugarcane, water melon, and màiméndōng juice) or the above-mentioned Zēng Yè Tāng for deeper-lying patterns. Puffiness as the result of Cold is caused by a lack of flow and an impaired fluid metabolism, which results in an abnormal retention of fluids. To treat such conditions, use Lǐ Zhōng Sǎn 理中散 or Wǔ Líng Sǎn 五苓散 in Tàiyáng Fǔ Syndromes, with ingredients like guìzhī, báizhú, and zéxiè. When Dampness causes diarrhea, this results in loose stools and minor diarrhea, as opposed to the symptom of "diarrhea with undigested food particles" (*sūn xiè* 飧泄) mentioned in the first section of this chapter.

As Gāo Shìzōng stresses, the five pathogenic factors described in this line are linked to the Five Dynamic Agents and to their influence on the human body, which in Gāo's interpretation of this line manifests directly in the state of the vessels.

* * *

Commentary by Gāo Shìzōng 高士宗

五行之氣，應於經脈，木氣為風，故風勝則經脈為之振動矣。火氣為熱，熱勝則經脈為之癰腫矣。癰腫為熱，與上文周身之寒腫不同也。金氣為燥，燥勝則經脈為之干枯矣。水氣為寒，寒勝則經脈如運樞之外浮矣。土氣為濕，濕勝則經脈為之濡潤而下瀉矣。

The Qì of the Five Dynamic Agents resonates in the channels and vessels: The Qì of Wood is Wind, and a predominance of Wood therefore results in shaking and trembling in the vessels! The Qì of Fire is Heat, and a predominance of Heat therefore results in swollen welling-abscesses in the vessels! Swollen welling-abscesses are hot, which means that this is not the same as the generalized Cold swelling mentioned above. The Qì of Metal is Parching, and a predominance of Parching therefore results in desiccation in the vessels! The Qì of Water is Cold, and a predominance of Cold therefore results in outward floating of the channels like a revolving pivot! The Qì of Earth is Dampness, and a predominance of Dampness therefore results in sogginess and drenching in the channels and then diarrhea!

* * *

WHETHER WE FOLLOW GĀO'S FAIRLY NARROW INTERPRETATION OF the pathologies (stirring, swelling, dryness, floating, and drenching outpouring) or read them as more general pathologies in the body, this line is thus the perfect example of the sort of cosmic "resonance" (*yìng* 應) that is the central topic of this text. Looking more closely at individual terms used in this passage, the character *dòng* 動 originally simply means "movement" and can be used in both a positive or a negative sense. In medical literature, it tends to carry a negative connotation. One common example is the phrase *tāi dòng* 胎動 "fetal stirring," which is translated in most TCM literature as "uterine contractions" but really refers to fetal unrest, i.e., abnormal activity of the fetus inside the uterus, and can be a warning sign for a threatened miscarriage. *Dòng* is also the term most commonly used to describe the activity of pathological Wind in the body, which causes the body to stir and shake in random, unpredictable, and sometimes harmful movements like seizures or spasms. Like an invasion of "bugs" (*chóng* 虫), which the Chinese character for "wind" includes in its character 風, Wind pathologies inside the body have the tendency to move around the body without a fixed location, appearing and disappearing unexpectedly like ants or cockroaches that hide in the rotten structures of an old house waiting for an opportunity to emerge and further weaken the victim before they go back into hiding. As so aptly stated in the "Discourse on Wind" in *Sù Wèn* Chapter 42 《風論》, "Wind is the leader of the hundred diseases" (*fēng zhě bǎi bìng zhī zhǎng yě* 風者百病之長也). For more information on this important pathology, see that chapter.

Another important concept in medical literature that is mentioned in this passage is *fú* 浮, which I have translated literally in the context of the present line as "floating" to avoid reading my own interpretation into the original statement. Scholars and clinicians throughout the ages have disagreed on the precise meaning of the term here. As the commentary by Zhāng Zhìcōng demonstrates, sometimes the term is read as referring to the spirit (and Qì) floating astray ("*Shén* and Qì then float"). More commonly, though, this term here is interpreted in the tradition of Wáng Bīng's reading as referring to puffy swelling, which is the result of an impeded circulation due to the stagnating influence of cold.

* * *

Commentary by Wáng Bīng 王冰

寒勝則陰氣結於玄府，玄府閉密，陽氣內攻，故為浮。

When Cold is predominant, Yīn Qì binds in the sweat pores, so the sweat pores are sealed shut. Yáng Qì attacks internally, and we therefore see floating."

* * *

What commentators do agree on is that "floating" here does not refer to a superficial quality of the pulse, as an inexperienced reader of this passage might be tempted to construe, based on the fact that *fú* is also a common descriptor of pulse quality.

A last term that requires a brief note is the phrase that I have translated literally as "drenching outpouring: *rú xiè* 濡瀉. Dr. Long interprets this compound here as soft stools that should be treated with formulas like Wèi Líng Tāng 胃苓湯 or Píng Wèi Sǎn 平胃散, to dry Dampness and activate the Stomach. While I generally hesitate to equate two Chinese terms that are written with distinct characters, in the case of diarrhea the characters 泄 and 瀉 are pronounced identically as *xiè* and are generally used interchangeably in early sources. In later medical literature, *xiè* 泄 tends to be used more often to refer to the pathology of diarrhea, while *xiè* 瀉 is used more frequently in the context of an intended treatment effect as "down-draining" of pathogenic factors like Cold, Fire, or Dampness to get rid of them.

Supporting my argument that they are here used interchangeably is the fact that an almost identical version of this line that is cited in *Sù Wèn* Chapter 71 《六元正紀大論》 uses the character 泄 instead of 瀉 (故風勝則動，熱勝則腫，燥勝則乾，寒勝則浮，濕勝則濡泄。) A third character, which is also pronounced *xiè* 洩, is generally accepted to be simply a scribal variation on 泄.

Section Five

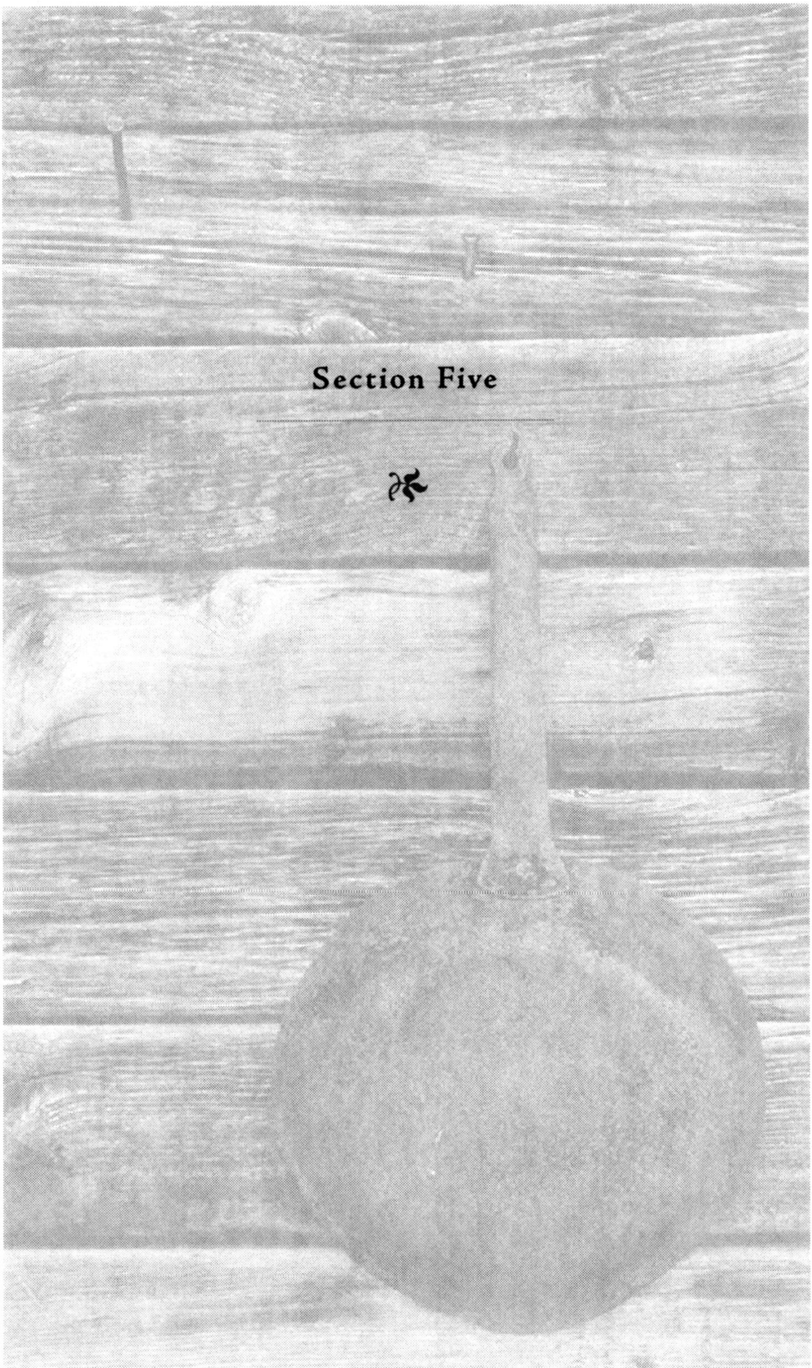

天有四時五行，以生長收藏，以生寒暑燥濕風。

人有五臟，化五氣，以生喜怒悲憂恐。

Tiān yǒu sì shí wǔ xíng,
yǐ shēng zhǎng shōu cáng,
yǐ shēng hán shǔ zào shī fēng.

Rén yǒu wǔ zàng, huà wǔ qì, yǐ
shēng xǐ nù bēi yōu kǒng.

In Heaven, there are the Four Seasons and Five Dynamic Agents. By means of these, birth, growth, harvest, and storage take place. By means of these, Cold, Summerheat, Parching, Dampness, and Wind are engendered.

In humans, there are the Five Zàng Organs, which transform the Five Qì and by means of these engender happiness, anger, grief, mourning, and fear.

Commentary by Zhāng Jièbīn 張介賓

四時者，春夏秋冬。五行者，木火土金水。合而言之，則春屬木而主生，其化以風；夏屬火而主長，其化以暑；長夏屬土而主化，其化以濕；秋屬金而主收，其化以燥；冬屬水而主藏，其化以寒。五行各一，惟火有君相之分。此言寒暑燥濕風者，即五行之化也。《五營運》等論言寒暑燥濕風火者，是為六氣也。。。

五臟者，心肺肝脾腎也。五氣者，五臟之氣也。由五氣以生五志。如本論及《五營運大論》，俱言心在志為喜，肝在志為怒，脾在志為思，肺在志為憂，腎在志為恐。

The Four Seasons are spring, summer, fall, and winter. The Five Dynamic Agents are Wood, Fire, Earth, Metal and Water. Speaking of these in combination, spring is associated with Wood and rules birth; its transformation occurs by Wind. Summer is associated with Fire and rules growth; its transformation occurs by Summerheat. Long Summer is associated with Earth and rules transformation; its transformation occurs by Dampness. Fall is associated with Metal and rules harvesting; its transformation occurs by Parching. Winter is associated with Water and rules storage; its transformation occurs by Cold. The Five Dynamic Agents each are one, with the sole exception of Fire being divided into Sovereign Fire (jūn huǒ 君火) and Ministerial Fire (xiàng huǒ 相火). This passage says that Cold, Summerheat, Parching, Dampness, and Wind are indeed the transformations of the Five Dynamic Agents. When discourses such as the ones on the Five Movements (i.e., Sù Wèn Chapter 67) speak of Cold, Summerheat, Parching, Dampness, Wind, and Fire, this is a reference to the Six Qì.

The Five Zàng Organs are Heart, Lung, Liver, Spleen and Kidney. The Five Qì are the Qì of the Five Zàng Organs. It is out of the Five Qì that the Five Wills are engendered. As the present Discourse and the Great Discourse on the Five Movements (i.e., Sù Wèn Chapter 67) both state, the Heart among the Wills is happiness, the Liver among the Wills is anger, the Spleen among the Wills is ruminating, the Lung among the Wills is mourning, and the Kidney among the Wills is fear.

THIS SECTION AGAIN EMPHASIZES THE CORRELATIONS AND interconnections between the external and the internal environment of the human body. In the first line, the four seasons in the macrocosm create a healthy normal response in the natural world, which is the cycle of life: giving birth in the spring, growing in the summer, gathering in the fall, and storage (in the sense of hibernation or of plants dropping or reducing their above-ground foliage and "hiding" underground to preserve their energy in the winter), before the cycle starts again in the following spring. Isn't it beautiful how this line resolves the apparent conflict between cycles of four and of five, with the Four Seasons associated with the natural processes, and the Five Dynamic Agents associated with the generation of the five climatic factors?

The four key terms to describe the seasons, *sheng* 生, *zhǎng* 長, *shōu* 收, and *cáng* 藏 are here translated in their most general sense, but it is important to remember that they each have a very specific meaning in the context of the seasonal cycle: *Shēng* 生 "birth" derives from the notion of "sprouting" as suggested by early versions of the character that literally depict a plant pushing up through the surface of the earth from underneath to form its first leaf.

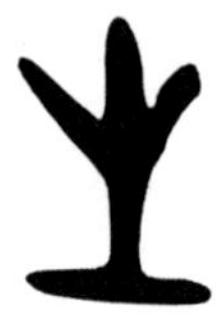
Early character for *Shēng* 生.

The earliest versions of the character for *zhǎng* 長 "to grow" or "to lengthen," depict a person with long hair. The character for *shōu* 收 "to harvest," is a combination of "threshing" with a hook- or sickle-like object. In a larger sense, it can mean "to receive" or "to gather in," and in the context of physiology or pharmacological action even to "draw inward," such as when it describes the process of Qì consolidation in a newborn baby. Finally, *cáng* 藏 "to store" or "to hide" (as in "to conceal in deep grass," suggested perhaps by the grass radical) can also mean "to go underground," which is what most animals and plants do to survive the harsh cold of winter, like a bear in hibernation.

The second half of this passage moves us directly back into the realm of the human body as the microcosm that operates within the same inherent cosmic structure and in resonance with the macrocosm. At this level, we have the Five *Zàng* Organs, which engender the Five

Wills (also known as Five Emotions, *wǔ qíng* 五情) by means of the "Five Qì." This brings us to one of the most difficult phrases in this section of the text, namely how to understand the phrase "transforms the Five Qì" (*huà wǔ qì* 化五氣), resulting in some substantial disagreement among commentators. As so often in this entire discourse, the precise meaning of Qì is left unexplained. Zhāng Jièbīn explains them in the quote cited above as the "Qì of the Five *Zàng* Organs" (五臟之氣), which in turn engender the Five Wills (*wǔ zhì* 五志). Zhāng Zhìcōng, on the other hand, explains them as the "Qì of the Five Dynamic Agents" (五行之氣). Rather than narrowing the meaning of the term by explanation and personal interpretation, as these two authors have done, the best approach, in my opinion, is to consciously try to embrace the ambiguity and multiplicity of meanings in the term Qì and contemplate both options. The original text is, after all, the direct manifestation of a perspective that truly sees the macrocosm and all its associated microcosms not only as correlated and resonating with each other, but perhaps as identical and intertwined in ways that we modern humans are unable to grasp other than in short moments when we can turn off our rational minds and perceive with our *Shén* instead. As such, it is perhaps the greatest challenge for any reader of the *Huáng Dì Nèi Jīng* to accept that these fine details ultimately do not matter, since each one is identical on some deep level with the others. To grasp the basic homology between processes that occur in the natural world, in the human realm of society, and inside the human body means to understand the basic identity between Heaven, Humanity, and Earth. It should be noted here, however, that the doctrine of Five Movements and Six Qì, which Zhāng Jièbīn alludes to in the commentary above, was not developed fully until many centuries after the composition of the original *Nèi Jīng* text, and we must therefore always be cautious about not reading such later theories back into the text.

Before moving on to the next line, readers familiar with the medical classics will recognize the Five Emotions or Wills and know to relate happiness to the Heart, anger to the Liver, mourning to the Lung, and fear to the Kidney. And as you may have noticed, the character here used for the emotion of the Spleen, namely *bēi* 悲, which

I have translated literally as "grief," is more often associated with the emotion of the Lung. The easiest explanation for this discrepancy here is to read *bēi* 悲 "grief" as a scribal error for *sī* 思 "ruminating," which is the standard emotion associated with the Spleen. This argument is supported by other lists of the Five Emotions and their associated *Zàng* Organs in the *Nèi Jīng*, including the description of the Spleen and its resonances. Another intriguing possibility is that this list here reflects an alternative conception of the Five Emotions in general, and of the way in which the Spleen-Stomach system is affected by them in particular. For another non-standard account of the effect of the emotions in the *Nèi Jīng* corpus, see this quotation from *Sù Wèn* Chapter 39:

Quotation from Sù Wèn[1]

百病生於氣也，怒則氣上，喜則氣緩，悲則氣消，恐則氣下，寒則氣收，炅則氣泄，驚則氣亂，勞則氣耗，思則氣結。

This is how the Hundred Diseases are engendered by Qì: Anger results in ascent of Qì, happiness in laxness of Qì, grief in diminishment of qì, fear in descent of Qì, Cold in drawing inward of Qì, fireheat in leakage of Qì, fright in disordering of Qì, taxation in expenditure of Qì, and ruminating in knotting of Qì.

While this passage does cite the standard list of anger, happiness, grief, and fear (presumably related to the Liver, Heart, Lung, and Kidney), it then adds a handful of other factors, before finishing with ruminating, as the emotion usually associated with the Spleen. It is not clear in this citation, however, whether these emotions are already associated with the *Zàng* Organs, as a modern reader would

[1] *Sù Wèn* 《素問》 Chapter 39, *Jǔ Tòng Lùn* 舉痛論 (Discourse on Lifting Pain).

assume, or whether they are simply listed as different facets of Qì that cause disease. Similarly, the important essay "Rooted in Spirit" in the *Líng Shū* 靈樞 (Divine Pivot) does not repeat the standard list but describes the pathological effect of emotional upheaval in this way:

* * *

Quotation from Líng Shū 靈樞 [2]

是故怵惕思慮者則傷神，神傷則恐懼流淫而不止。因悲哀動中者，竭絕而失生。喜樂者，神憚散而不藏。愁憂者，氣閉塞而不行。盛怒者，迷惑而不治。恐懼者，神蕩憚而不收。

For this reason, rumination and discernment [with] alarm and anxiety result in injury to the Shén. When the Shén is injured, fear and panic flow without restraint or stopping. Stirring of the center because of grief and sorrow mean exhaustion and interrupted flow, and then loss of life. Happiness and joy make the Shén frightened and scattered so that it is no longer stored. Gloominess and worry block and congest the Qì, preventing it from moving freely. Exuberant anger leads to confusion and delusion and to a lack of good order. Fear and panic rattle and frighten away the Shén instead of gathering it in.

* * *

As Elisabeth Hsu has suggested in the article cited above on "Outward Form and Inward Qi," these different accounts of the emotions might point to an earlier conception of the body that was either dualistic, following the Yīn-Yáng model by contrasting happiness, associated with the Heart as the representative of the upper body, and anger, associated with the Liver and the lower body, or perhaps trifold, with the addition of the Lung, as seen in *Líng Shū* Chapter 66. There, anger is still the emotion of the Liver, but the Heart is associated with

[2] *Líng Shū* 《靈樞》 Chapter 8, *Běn Shén* 本神 (Rooted in Spirit).

yōu sī 憂思 "mourning and ruminating."[3] One possible explanation for that conundrum may be suggested by Wáng Bīng's commentary on the following line in the present text: He explains the correlation of anger with injury to Yīn, and of happiness with injury to Yáng by stating that anger causes the Qì to rise, and sudden ascent of Qì means injury to Yīn. Contrary to what we tend to think in Western psychology, Wáng then goes on to state that happiness causes the Qì to move down, and sudden descent of Qì injures Yáng (怒則氣上，喜則氣下，故暴卒氣上則傷陰，暴卒氣下則傷陽). If we read happiness here in this medical context as the emotion associated with the Heart and the upper body and, in the case of pathology, with causing Qì to fall, we might be able to appreciate Wáng Bīng's explanation a little more easily.

[3] Hsu, "Outward Form and Inward Body," 108-109.

故喜怒傷氣，寒暑傷形。
暴怒傷陰，暴喜傷陽。

Gù xǐ nù shāng qì, hán shǔ shāng xíng.
Bào nù shāng yīn, bào xǐ shāng yáng.

This being so, happiness and anger injure the Qì; Cold and Summerheat injure the Form; fulminant anger injures Yīn; fulminant happiness injures Yáng.

Commentary by Gāo Shìzōng 高士宗

人之志意起於內，故喜怒傷氣；天之邪氣起於外，
故寒暑傷形。舉喜怒而悲憂恐在其中，舉寒暑而燥濕風在其中。
在天則寒為陰，暑為陽，在人則怒為陰，喜為陽。故卒暴而怒，
則傷吾身之陰氣；卒暴而喜，則傷吾身之陽氣。

People's emotions arise on the inside; hence happiness and anger injure the Qì. Heaven's Evil Qì arise on the outside; hence Cold and Summerheat injure the Form. The text [only] mentions happiness and anger, but grief, worry, and fear are included among these as well; it [only] mentions Cold and Summerheat, but Parching, Dampness, and Wind are included among these as well. In Heaven then, Cold is Yīn and Summerheat is Yáng; in humans, anger is Yīn and happiness is Yáng. Therefore, sudden explosions of anger injure the body's Yīn Qì, while sudden explosions of happiness injure the body's Yáng Qì.

Continuing the train of thought from the previous section, this line contrasts the pathological effects of the external five climatic factors on the Form with the effects of the internal Five Emotions on the Qì. It is generally accepted, as stated explicitly in Gāo Shìzōng's commentary, that "happiness and anger" stand here for all the Five Emotions mentioned in the previous line, and that "Cold and Summerheat" imply not just these two but all climatic factors, hence including Dryness, Dampness, and Wind.

The contrast between emotional factors, which injure the Qì, and climatic factors, that injure the Form, makes sense when we consider that the emotions arise internally and therefore primarily injure the Qì in the interior of the body. The climatic factors, on the other hand, affect the body in the exterior layer first, entering through the skin and body hair to then penetrate more deeply into the flesh, network vessels, and finally into the internal organs. It is not difficult to imagine the clinical importance of this distinction between internal emotional and external climatic causes of disease and their effect on the Qì and Form, respectively. To cite just one example, the skilled practitioner is able to diagnostically determine in a complex disease case whether the patient is suffering primarily from disorder in the Qì or in the Form. On the basis of this knowledge, she or he will know clearly whether the primary disease cause is an internal one or an external one. And the stratagem that "To treat disease, you must seek it in the basics," will then indicate the direction that treatment should take to ensure maximum efficacy.

Despite this neat and convincing distinction between internal causes affecting the Qì and external causes affecting the Form, the statement that Cold and Summerheat injure the Form does contradict an earlier line (see Section Four, page 107) that "Cold injures the Form; Heat harms the Qì" (寒傷形，熱傷氣). What are we to make of this contradiction in understanding the effect of external pathogens on the human body in clinical terms? Once again, we have to stretch our minds and accept that Yīn and Yáng can be witnessed at many different levels of the macrocosm and the microcosm of the body, sometimes at the same time, and that they will invariably contradict each other at times. So we do not simply have the neat effects of pure Yīn versus pure Yáng to reckon with, as some of these apparently simple lines in the *Nèi Jīng* might suggest at first sight, whether we are dealing with food or weather or any other number of factors. Rather, the messy reality of our complex internal and external lives transcends a neat Yīn-Yáng division, forcing us to consider the Yáng aspect of Yīn and the Yīn aspect of Yáng, with mutually interacting and often contradictory effects at the same time. And of course then we have to differentiate which of the Yīn and Yáng aspects of the body are responding internally in which way to a complex onslaught of factors from the outside and vice versa. The following section of the text hence looks at "extreme/double Yīn" and "extreme/double Yáng" as most likely a combination of internal and external pathologies.

* * *

Commentary by Zhāng Jièbīn 張介賓

氣為陽，血為陰。肝藏血，心藏神。暴怒則肝氣逆而血亂，故傷陰。暴喜則心氣緩而神逸，故傷陽。如《行針篇》曰：多陽者多喜，多陰者多怒。亦各從其類也。

Qì is Yáng, Blood is Yīn. The Liver stores the Blood, and the Heart stores the Shén. Fulminant Anger results in countercurrent flow of Liver Qì and then in chaos in the Blood. Hence it injures Yīn. Fulminant happiness results in laxness of the Heart Qì, and in the escape of the Shén. Hence it injures Yáng. As the Líng Shū chapter on Needling states: "A lot of Yáng means a lot of happiness. A lot of Yīn means a lot of anger." This is also a case of each conforming with its category.

* * *

Elaborating on our discussion of the reasons why anger is associated with Yīn and happiness with Yáng, the *Lèi Jīng* commentary explains that anger is the emotion associated with the Liver, and when the Qì of anger disrupts the physiological functioning of the Liver, it is no longer able to store Blood. Instead of being stored, it flows chaotically and thereby is a manifestation of injury to Yīn. By contrast, happiness is associated with the Heart, which is in charge of storing and anchoring the *Shén*. Happiness has the effect of relaxing the Qì of the Heart and hence causing the *Shén* to escape, thereby injuring Yáng. It is interesting to note the twist here in the last sentence, identified as a quotation from *Líng Shū* Chapter 67, which seems to imply almost the opposite of the statement in *Sù Wèn* Chapter 5. The context there makes it clear that the phrases "a lot of Yáng" and "a lot of Yīn" in this chapter are references to patients with a predominance of Yáng or Yīn, and that the finding of a lot of anger or happiness is meant to assist the physician in classifying patients as either Yīn or Yáng types. In other words, *Líng Shū* 靈樞 Chapter 67 associates the expression of happiness with a person who is mostly

Yáng, and of anger with a Yīn type, while *Sù Wèn* Chapter 5 appears to do the opposite, namely associating happiness with injury to Yáng and anger with injury to Yīn. One possible explanation for this seeming contradiction might be that *Líng Shū* Chapter 67 is discussing the physiological expression of happiness or anger, while *Sù Wèn* Chapter 5 is talking about a great pathological excess, as suggested by the word "fulminant." That is apparently the direction Zhāng Zhìcóng is suggesting with his commentary:

* * *

Commentary by Zhāng Zhìcōng 張志聰

多陽者多喜；多陰者多怒，喜屬陽而怒屬陰也。是以卒暴而怒，
則有傷於陰矣；卒暴之喜，則有傷於陽矣。

The reason why a lot of Yáng means a lot of happiness and a lot of Yīn means a lot of anger is that happiness is associated with Yáng, and anger is associated with Yīn. For this reason, sudden fulminant anger results in injury to the Yīn [aspect of the body]! Sudden fulminant happiness results in injury to the Yáng [aspect of the body]!

* * *

厥氣上行，滿脈去形。

Jué qì shàng xíng,
mǎn mài qù xíng.

Reversal Qì moves upward,
filling the vessels
and leaving the Form.

Commentary by Wáng Bīng 王冰

逆氣上行，滿於經絡，則神氣浮越，去離形骸矣。

When countercurrent Qì moves upward and fills the channels and network vessels, Shén Qì floats astray and departs from the Form and the bones!

Commentary by Zhāng Zhìcōng 張志聰

陰陽之氣厥逆上行，則五臟之氣滿於脈而離脫于真藏之形矣。
此言寒暑傷在外形身之陰陽，喜怒傷於內藏氣之陰陽也。
張兆璜曰：傷陽則氣厥於上。傷陰則血滿於脈。

When the Qì of Yīn and Yáng reverse direction and flow upward against the current, the Qì of the Five Zàng Organs fills up the vessels and departs from the Form in the True Zàng Organs. This passage states that injury from Cold and Summerheat affects the Yīn and Yáng of the outside Form, while Elation and Anger injure the Yīn and Yáng of the internally stored Qì. Zhāng Zhàohuáng says: "Injury to the Yáng results in Qì reversing direction into the upper body. Injury to the Yīn results in Blood filling the vessels."

There are two ways to read this line, as exemplified by the quotations cited here. We can follow the lead of Wáng Bīng, as cited above, and interpret the fullness in the vessels as the result of a pathological upward flow of Qì in a countercurrent direction. This fullness in the channels, due to the upward flow of Qì, causes the more subtle *shén* qì to depart from the physical body.

Alternatively, we can read the countercurrent flow of Qì here as the effect of injury to Yáng, and the fullness in the vessels as the parallel, but not related, effect of injury to Yīn.

The commentary by Zhāng Zhìcōng appears to embrace both options: First Zhāng himself explains that Qì filling the vessels and leaving the Form is the direct effect of both Yīn Qì and Yáng Qì rising into the upper body contrary to their normal physiological flow. Then, however, he goes on to cite another commentator who reads the second half of this line as referring not to the result of the first half but as an altogether different pathology, one associated with injury to Yīn as opposed to injury to Yáng.

* * *

Commentary by Zhāng Jièbīn 張介賓

厥，逆也。言寒暑喜怒之氣，暴逆於上，則陽獨實，故滿脈。
陽亢則陰離，故去形。此孤陽之象也。
《脈經》曰：諸浮脈無根者死，有表無裡者死，其斯之謂。

Reversal means countercurrent flow. This passage states that when the Qì of Cold and Summerheat and of happiness and anger moves fulminantly upward in a countercurrent direction, this results in Yáng alone becoming replete, hence filling up the vessels. A hyperactivity of Yáng results in Yīn leaving and therefore departing from the Form. This is the image of solitary Yáng. The Pulse Classic says: 'All floating pulses that lack a root mean death. Presence in the exterior and absence in the interior means death.' This is what this passage means.

* * *

Nì 逆 and *jué* 厥 are two characters with similar meanings that are, however, distinguished by context and subtle connotations in

Chinese medical literature and therefore need to be translated differently. Teasing out this difference may help us make sense of this line: *Nì* 逆 has two meanings in classical Chinese literature: Advancing to meet somebody (friend or foe) head on; and going against the stream, flow, or current. By extension, it can refer to any contrary movement or action, from retrograde planets to rebellion and disobedience, or just action contrary to rules or convention. In medical literature, it refers to a pathological movement of Qì that is contrary to its healthy direction, especially in the context of the movement of *Zàng* Organ Qì. Hence Wiseman and most other translators render it as "counterflow." To express the important notion that this *nì* type of flow always moves against the prevailing, normal, and physiological flow (expressed by the term *shùn* 順 meaning "flowing along with the current"), I have chosen the stronger "countercurrent" to translate *nì* in the present book. In the medical classics, the term *nì* is associated with an unhealthy movement of Qì or fluids that tends to runs upward into the upper body and is most common in the compounds "countercurrent ascent of Stomach Qì" (*wèi qì shàng nì* 胃氣上逆) and "countercurrent ascent of Lung Qì" (*fèi qì shàng nì* 肺氣上逆), but can also refer to the upward rushing of depressed and pent up Liver Qì. Note that it is in all these cases associated with a pathological movement that goes upward, contrary to the natural downward movement or, in the case of the Liver, in excess of its healthy effusing and dispersing action. In other contexts, *nì* can refer to an unfavorable turn in the disease dynamic, away from a movement towards recovery and health. In both meanings, it is contrasted with *shùn* 順 "flow in the proper direction." In terms of its etymology, the original character 屰 depicts a big person, a person with arms spread out (大), who is turned upside down, with the radical for "movement" 辶 added later. In the *Shuō Wén Jiě Zì* dictionary, it is explained as *yíng* 迎 "to meet/welcome somebody."

Used less commonly and in a narrower meaning, *jué* 厥 is often translated as "loss of consciousness" or "fainting," especially in modern TCM literature and in non-medical dictionaries. While this interpretation may be an accurate reflection of its standard use in modern Chinese and in contemporary medical writings, in classical sources and more specialized contexts it can be misleading since it narrows a description of Qì flow down to the most dramatic clinical manifestation thereof. Strictly speaking, *jué* refers to a dangerous disruption of the Qì flow that leads to such dramatic symptoms as fainting when it involves a clouding of the Heart. In this more specific sense of a critical sudden blockage of healthy flow, it can also be used in phrases like "Reversal Cold in the four extremities" *sì zhī jué lěng* 四肢厥冷, where it has nothing to do with fainting, or even in the name of the Liver channel: Jué Yīn "Reverting Yīn." In classical medical literature, it thus refers to a serious condition where the natural flow is stopped, with the result that it reverses direction. Looking at its etymology, it is a combination of 厂 (meaning "precipice") and 欮, an old character meaning "hiccup," which is identified as the phonetic, but must also have been chosen for its meaning. That character, *jué* 欮, in turn consists of the "big person turned upside down" that we have already encountered in the character for 逆, in combination with *qiàn* 欠, meaning "shortness of breath."

Returning to our discussion of the passage from *Sù Wèn* Chapter 5 above and the meaning of "Reversal Qì moves upward," why does the text use *jué* Reversal here instead of the more common *nì* "countercurrent"? In my reading, *jué* stands out for its association with a more drastic, sudden, and often obfuscating blockage of Qì flow, which fits perfectly with the previous line that discusses "fulminant anger" and "fulminant happiness." Both of these pathologies strike me as prime candidates for exactly this sort of a drastic physical response.

喜怒不節，寒暑過度，生乃不固。

故重陰必陽，重陽必陰。

故曰：冬傷於寒，春必溫病；春傷於風，夏生飧泄；夏傷於暑，
秋必痎瘧；秋傷於濕，冬生咳嗽。

Xǐ nù bù jié, hán shǔ guò dù,
shēng nǎi bù gù.

Gù chóng/zhòng yīn bì yáng,
Chóng/zhòng yáng bì yīn.

Gù yuē: Dōng shāng yú hán,
chūn bì wēn bìng; chūn shāng yú fēng,
xià shēng sūn xiè; xià shāng yú shǔ,
qiū bì jiē nüè; qiū shāng yú shī,
dōng shēng ké sòu.

When happiness and anger
are not duly measured,
when Cold and Summerheat
exceed the norm, life is then not secure.

Therefore, extreme/double Yīn
must become Yáng;
extreme/double Yáng must become Yīn.

Therefore it is said:
"Cold injury in winter invariably
results in Warm Disease in the spring;
Wind injury in the spring will
produce diarrhea with undigested food
particles in the summer; Summerheat
injury in the summer invariably
results in malaria in the autumn;
Dampness injury in the autumn
will produce cough in the winter."

With this passage, we again encounter the potent dynamic of Yīn and Yáng transforming into each other when they have reached a pivotal (or "double") state of extreme development. This dynamic of each aspect turning into its opposite lies at the heart of the Chinese world view, whether in physiology or pathology, or in any other macrocosmic and microcosmic cycle. It is literally the mechanism that "makes the world go 'round." One of the earliest demonstrations of this same principle is the interpretation and behavior of the lines in the 64 hexagrams of the *Yì Jīng* 易經 (Classic of Changes). Briefly, each hexagram is built by stacking up six lines, which are either Yīn or Yáng. In the three-coin-toss method, these lines are created by tossing three coins and interpreting the resulting combination of heads and tails as a Yīn or Yáng line in four different variations. Three heads make an "old" and therefore changing Yīn line, while three tails make an "old" Yáng line. Two heads and one tail make a static or "young" Yáng line, while two tails and a head make a static Yīn line. The point here is that the "old" lines, the ones that are either pure Yīn or pure Yáng are read as unstable "changing" lines, in the sense of being about to flip into their opposite, while combinations of Yīn and Yáng results are interpreted as stable.

As already stated above, we can read the character 重 either as *chóng*, in which case it means "double" or "repeated" in the sense of one layer piled upon another layer, or as *zhòng*, which literally means "heavy" but could here mean "serious" or "substantial." I personally like to read it as *chóng* ("double") here, in the sense of a situation where a person is exposed to not just one Yīn or Yáng factor, but to a combination of two, since the previous line explicitly states the danger of both internal and external pathologies, namely the emotions in addition to seasonal factors. As a result, the person experiencing this constellation develops a pathology because the system gets overwhelmed by too much of either Yīn or Yáng. Mǎ Shì's explanation clearly refers to a doubling up of Yīn or Yáng, such as exposure to Cold in a Yīn season or exposure to Cold in a Yáng season.

Commentary by Mǎ Shì 馬蒔[4]

何以見寒暑不可過度也?蓋時之屬陰者，而復感於寒，則重陰必陽，熱證乃作。時之屬陽者，而復感於熱，則重陽必陰，寒病乃生。

試觀冬傷於寒，寒毒藏於肌膚，至春當為溫病。春傷於風，風氣通於肝，肝邪有餘，來侮脾土，留連至夏，當為飧泄之證。夏傷於暑，暑汗不出，至秋涼風相薄，而為寒熱往來之瘧。秋傷於濕，則濕蒸而為熱，熱者火也，火乘肺金而至冬，寒與熱搏，當為欬嗽之證。故即春夏之病，則重陽必陰之義可識矣;即秋冬之病，則重陰必陽之義可識矣。

Why is it that we must not exceed the proper measure in exposure to Cold or Summerheat? In the seasons that are associated with Yīn, if we additionally contract Cold, double Yīn invariably turns into Yáng. This is how Heat patterns are produced. In the seasons that are associated with Yáng, if we additionally contract Heat, double Yáng invariably turns into Yīn, and this is how Cold disease is engendered.

Let us look at being injured by Cold in winter: This Cold poison is stored in the skin and, when spring arrives, becomes Warm Disease. If there is injury from Wind in the spring, the Qì of Wind communicates with the Liver, and when there is excess evil in the Liver, it insults Spleen Earth. Lingering all the way until summer, it then produces the pattern of diarrhea with undigested food particles. If there is injury from Summerheat in the summer and the Summerheat sweat fails to exit, when autumn arrives it will get entangled with Cool Wind, which produces malaria of intermittent Cold and Heat. If there is injury from Dampness in autumn, the Dampness can smolder and turn into Heat. This Heat is Fire. The Fire overwhelms Lung Metal, and when winter arrives, the Cold and Heat strike each other, causing the pattern of cough. As such, from these precise illnesses in spring and summer, we can know the meaning of 'double Yáng must turn into Yīn'; from these precise

[4] Mǎ Shì 馬蒔 *Huáng Dì Nèi Jīng Sù Wèn Zhù Zhèng Fā Wéi* 《黃帝內經素問注証發微》 (The Yellow Emperor's Inner Classic, Plain Questions Annotated, Verified, and Explored in Detail), 1586.

illnesses in autumn and winter, we can know the meaning of 'double Yīn must turn into Yáng.'

* * *

I WOULD LIKE TO OFFER ANOTHER POSSIBILITY TO CONSIDER IN READING this line, one that is suggested by the context of the chapter: "Double" could here also refer not just to a doubling up of seasonal Yīn or Yáng with additional external Cold or Heat, respectively, whether from extreme exposure to weather or improper clothing, but to a pathological combination of external Yīn or Yáng with internal Yīn or Yáng, whether from diet, as in the discussion of Flavor and Qì above, or from emotions, as suggested in the statement in above that fulminant anger injures the Yīn while fulminant happiness injures the Yáng. This line of thinking is supported by the introductory passage of this section, which explicitly juxtaposes internal and external factors as the reason why life is no longer secure. By contrast, the following commentary by Wáng Bīng appears to advocate a reading of 重 as *zhòng* in the meaning of "serious."

* * *

Commentary by Wáng Bīng 王冰

傷於四時之氣，皆能為病。以傷寒為毒者，最為殺厲之氣，中而即病，故曰傷寒；不即病者，寒毒藏於肌膚至春變為溫病，至夏變為暑病。故養生者，必慎傷於邪也。風中于表則內應於肝，肝氣乘脾，故飧泄。生氣通天論云：春傷于風，邪氣留連，乃為洞泄。夏暑已甚，秋熱復壯，兩熱相攻，故為痎瘧。秋濕既多，冬水復王，水濕相得，肺氣又衰，故冬寒甚則為嗽。

Injury from the Qì of any of the four seasons can equally cause disease. If the poisoning agent is Cold Damage, in the most extreme circumstances this is the Qì of Lethal Pestilence. This is called "Cold Damage" if patients immediately fall ill after being struck. If they do not immediately fall ill, the Cold poison is stored in the skin and flesh and transforms into Warm Disease when spring arrives, or into Summerheat Disease when summer arrives. This is the reason why those who nurture life invariably pay close attention to injury from evil [Qì]. When Wind strikes the Exterior, it resonates internally with the Liver. Because Liver Qì overwhelms the Spleen, we see diarrhea with undigested food particles. As the "Discourse on Vital Qì Connecting Freely with Heaven" (Sù Wèn Chapter 3) states: "If a person is injured by Wind in the spring, the evil Qì can linger and continue, which eventually results in throughflux diarrhea." If the Heat in the summer is already great, and the Heat of autumn is again very strong, these two forms of Heat attack each other, hence producing malaria. If the Dampness of autumn is already profuse, and then again the Water of winter is effulgent, Water and Dampness gang up together, and Lung Qì is weakened further. For this reason, great Cold in the winter produces cough.

* * *

LASTLY, A BRIEF NOTE IS IN ORDER TO SHED LIGHT ON THE PHRASE "Dampness injury in the autumn" (*qiū shāng yú shī* 秋傷於濕): Some commentators explain this unusual association of autumn with Dampness here as a textual error and suggest replacing it with *zào* 燥 (parching), its precise opposite. Given that autumn and the Lung are generally associated with dryness, this would make good clinical sense. Other scholars attempt to make sense of this phrase as written from a medical perspective by explaining that Dampness in the autumn encumbers the Spleen and Stomach and impairs the Lung function of "depurative downbearing" (*sù jiàng* 肅降), so that Qì rises against the current instead, causing cough in winter.

Regardless of how one reads this phrase, the main idea to take away from this section of the text, in my eyes, is the equal importance of internal factors and external factors in the formation of disease. The need to moderate and balance the emotions, and the clinical potential for diagnosing and treating an emotional imbalance and its physiological effects through the paradigm of the Five Dynamic Agents and *Zàng* Organs, are fundamental aspects of Chinese medicine that distinguish it from biomedicine and offer an effective perspective for any medical practitioner. While we may not like the fact that happiness is included as a pathogenic factor among the Five Emotions (more on this below), it is worth contemplating the wisdom of the ancients and their ideal of equanimity and detachment, in order to respond spontaneously and flexibly to the Dào of the universe. This ideal is expressed in numerous places throughout the *Nèi Jīng*.

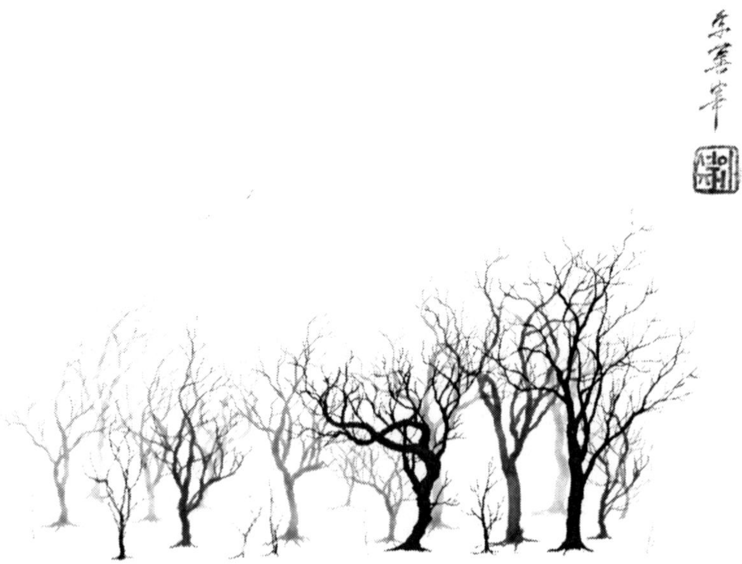

Quotation from Líng Shū 靈樞[5]

故智者之養生也，必順四時而適寒暑，和喜怒而安居處，節陰陽而調剛柔。如是則僻邪不至，長生久視。

As such, those with wisdom nurture life in this way: They invariably align themselves with the four seasons and adapt to Cold and Summerheat; harmonize their happiness and anger and make their living circumstances peaceful; and regulate Yīn and Yáng and attune hardness and softness. By acting like this, they make sure that deviation and evil do not arrive, and they lengthen their life and make their vision enduring.

Commentary by Z'ev Rosenberg

One of the most powerful therapeutic principles of Chinese medicine is the interface between the emotions and physiology. In modern medicine, one of the cutting-edge disciplines is called "psycho-neuro-immunology" (PNI), but this type of interactivity has been known in Chinese medicine since the Hàn Dynasty and before. In her excellent survey of early Hàn dynasty medicine *Pulse Diagnosis in Early Chinese Medicine* (Cambridge University Press, 2010), Elisabeth Hsu speaks about the "sentimental body." This is a conceptualization of the relationship between the emotions, Qì, and the *Zàng* organs as discussed in sections such as *Sù Wèn* Chapter 39. As she points out, "viscera gained prominence in medical language, because they were conceived as the seat of emotion, and as storage places of Qì (dynamics of which related

[5] *Líng Shū* 《靈樞》 Chapter 8.

to emotional processes)."[6] Here is a key passage (translated by Sabine Wilms), part of which has already been quoted above but which is important enough to be cited here at length:

Quotation from Sù Wèn[7]

帝曰：善。余知百病生於氣也，怒則氣上，喜則氣緩，
悲則氣消，恐則氣下，寒則氣收，炅則氣泄，驚則氣亂，
勞則氣耗，思則氣結，九氣不同，何病之生？

岐伯曰：怒則氣逆，甚則嘔血及飧泄，故氣上矣。

喜則氣和志達，榮衛通利，故氣緩矣。

悲則心系急，肺布葉舉，而上焦不通，榮衛不散，熱氣在中，故氣消矣。

恐則精卻，卻則上焦閉，閉則氣還，還則下焦脹，故氣不行矣。

The Emperor said: "Excellent! I know that the Hundred Diseases are engendered by Qì, with anger resulting in ascent of Qì, happiness resulting in laxness of Qì, grief resulting in the disintegration of Qì, fear resulting in descent of Qì, Cold resulting in constriction of Qì, fireheat resulting in leakage of Qì, fright resulting in disordering of Qì, taxation resulting in expenditure of Qì, and ruminating in knotting of Qì. Given these difference between the nine types of Qì, what kind of diseases do they engender?"

Qí Bó said: "Anger causes the Qì to move counterflow. In severe cases, this results in vomiting blood and diarrhea with undigested food particles. Thus [we say] 'ascent of Qì'.

[6] Hsu, Elisabeth, Pulse Diagnosis in Early Chinese Medicine, Cambridge University Press, Cambridge, U.K., 2010, 14.

[7] *Sù Wèn* 《素問》 Chapter 39.

Happiness makes the Qì harmonious and the Will untrammeled, and causes Yíng Provisioning and Wèi Defense to move about freely. Thus [we say] 'laxness of Qì'.

Grief makes the ties of the Heart tense. The Lung spreads out and its lobes are raised, movement in the Upper Jiāo is stopped, Yíng Provisioning and Wèi Defense are not distributed, and Heat Qì is present in the center. Thus we say 'disintegration of Qì'.

Fear causes the Essence to retreat, which causes blockage in the Upper Jiāo. This in turn makes the Qì turn around, causing distention in the Lower Jiāo. Thus we say 'failure of Qì to move [downwards]'".

* * *

We see here that emotions are a specific form of Qì that mobilize movement in the viscera, channels, and bodily structures. And this template allows us to understand how unregulated emotions can damage one's health. A clinical example that stands out for me from thirty years ago was a forty-year-old woman who had just moved from Tucson to Denver in the late summer. All of a sudden, she contracted a severe *chuǎn* 喘 asthmatic condition, with difficult breathing and coughing up of green phlegm, also indicating Liver/Gallbladder involvement. She was using a steroidal inhaler. I diagnosed a Wood-Metal disharmony, and gave her a modification of Wēn Dǎn Tāng 溫膽湯 (Warm the Gallbladder Decoction). I also asked her what type of events had occurred at the time she got sick, as she seemed emotionally "stuck," and had a straight-ahead stare in her eyes. She said, "oh, nothing at all." I pointed out that in my experience, it was rare to contract asthma in the summertime in the Southwestern deserts! She came back the following week, and I asked her again what had happened to her in the summer. She answered: "Oh, nothing much. My sixteen-year-old son drowned while swimming in a lake in July, and the following month my husband divorced me." I replied, "nothing much? Did you grieve for the loss of both your son and your marriage?" She answered, "no, I just moved up to Denver and started over." So you can see how she suppressed her grief and how this manifested as a physical disease instead.

Part Two

Resonances of the Five Directions in the Human Body

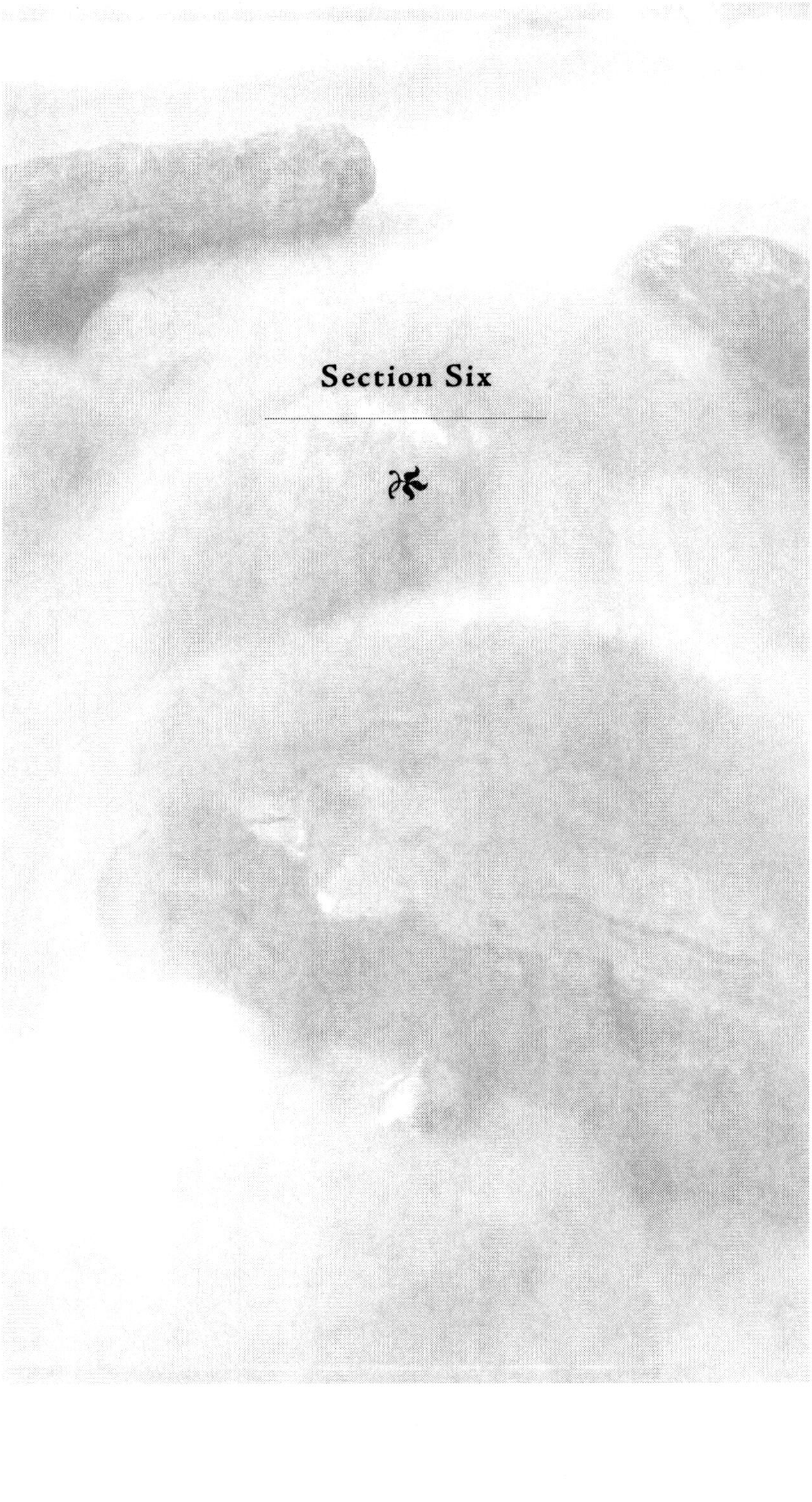

Section Six

帝曰：余聞上古聖人，論理人形，
列別臟腑，端絡經脈。

Dì yuē:
Yú wén shàng gǔ shèng rén,
lùn lǐ rén xíng, liè bié zàng fǔ,
duān luò jīng mài.

The Emperor said:
I have heard that the sages of high antiquity discussed and patterned the human body in accordance with deeper organizing principles, arrayed and differentiated the Zàng and Fǔ Organs, and laid out the channels and vessels in a grid of vertical stems and horizontal branches.

With this section, the Great Discourse shifts the discussion to a new topic, which we might regard as the core of the entire text: the detailed and often-cited descriptions of the resonances of the Five Dynamic Agents in Heaven, in the human body, and on Earth. To be sure, the statement above is not an easy section to make sense of, and there is a lot of disagreement among commentators on what exactly certain terms or phrases mean. Unfortunately, we are unable at this point to resolve these questions with certainty. For this reason, all I can do as a conscientious translator and scholar is to introduce the reader to some of the controversies and explain my reasoning for the choices I have made, always with the caveat that this is merely the reading that makes most sense to me personally, based on my understanding of the historical and cultural context, the etymology of characters and their use in general and in medical literature of this period, and related passages that may help us shed light on the present text.

In the Yellow Emperor's introduction to the question that he poses in the following section below, we already encounter some difficult terms. The first character in need of some explanation is *lǐ* 理: As suggested by the jade radical 玉, the character originally refers to the fine texture lines in jade. On a more abstract level, the character also refers to the principle, internal structural order, or any other type of inherent pattern that allows us to see a higher truth or structure behind the superficial appearance of a thing or concept. In my experience, *lǐ* 理 is one of those tricky characters in literary Chinese for which it is impossible to find a single English equivalent that works even just in all medical contexts, much less in philosophical or literary texts. In some contexts, something like "guiding principle" is an acceptable choice, while "pattern" works in others. In the present context, I read *lùnlǐ* 論理 as a combination of two verbs and have therefore chosen the wordy translation of "to pattern... in accordance with deeper organizing principles."

Likewise, the next phrase in this section to require an explanation is a combination of two characters that function as verbs: *duān luò* 端絡. *Duān* 端 originally depicts a plant growing straight up out of the soil, and can hence convey the idea of the very beginning, the sprouting, as well

會通六合，各從其經；氣穴所發，各有處名；溪谷屬骨，皆有所起；
分部逆從，各有條理；四時陰陽，盡有經紀；外內之應，皆有表裡。
其信然乎？

Huì tōng liù hé, gě cóng qí jīng;
qì xué suǒ fā, gè yǒu chù míng, xī gǔ shǔ
gǔ, jiē yǒu suǒ qǐ; fēn bù nì cóng,
gè yǒu tiáo lǐ; sì shí yīn yáng, jìn yǒu
jīng jì; wài nèi zhī yìng, jiē yǒu biǎo lǐ.

Qí xìn rán hū?

The intersecting and interconnected Six Matchings: they each follow their own Channels. The places where the Qì holes come to the surface: they each have their location and name. The attachments of the 'ravines' and 'valleys' [of the flesh] to the bone: they each have their starting point. The spatial divisions and specific sections for the coming and going [of Qì]: they each have their arrangements and organizing principles. The Four Seasons and Yīn and Yáng: they entirely have their warp and weft. The resonances between inside and outside: they all have their exterior and interior.

Is this something that is trustworthy?

as extremity, the far end of things, or the entirety and continuity between these two concepts. I am reading it here, however, in the sense of *zhī* 直 as "straight" or "vertical," a line or entity that goes straight up from the ground, which is an alternate meaning of this character. Luò 絡 refers to threads, often with the implied idea that they link up horizontally with other threads to form a network, as in the medical compound *jīng luò* 經絡 "channels and network vessels." In the particular combination and context of the present line, the two characters must mean something like "to form a net, or structural system, with main vertical lines and horizontal branches," which makes perfect sense here from a clinical perspective.

Next it must be pointed out that the separation in my layout of the text between the first and section sections is based more on convenience, ease of reading, the rhythm of the sentence, and my intuition than on clear grammar. You are free to disagree with it and read these two sections as a single sentence. Specifically, my reasoning is based on the fact that the rhythm, at least in my reading, shifts from short four-character combinations of two-character verbs with two-character objects in the first section to eight-character phrases that combine four-character topics with a four-character comments about them in the second section.

At the beginning of the second section, we encounter what is probably the most controversial term in this passage, namely *liù hé* 六合, which I have translated as "Six Matchings." The precise meaning of this compound here is an issue long debated by scholars. To reflect the linguistic directness of the Chinese term, I have finally settled on the translation of *hé* 合 as "matchings" after first considering translating it as "coordinates" in the sense of the following definition from the Concise Encyclopedia Brittanica: "Arrangement of reference lines or curves used to identify the location of points in space."[1] While this choice was appealing to me for its elegance, especially as we can then apply it to the system of channels and network vessels in the body, it introduces a way of thinking about spatial distribution that over-interprets the meaning of the original. Rather we should think of

[1] Encyclopaedia Brittanica: www.britannica.com/topic/coordinate-system, Nov. 6, 2017.

the compound more literally in the sense of "perfect match" or "pair," with the connotation that the outcome of such a perfect match or union is what delineates intellectually perceivable reality from what transcends it, as the following discussion will show. In the most direct and original sense of the character, its etymology suggests the meaning of a lid that covers or closes off a container. From this basic meaning, the character comes to mean "to conjoin," "to match," or even "to unite" or "to blend," such as in sexual intercourse (*hé yīn yáng* 合陰陽 "uniting Yīn and Yáng") or in "compounding medicinals" (*hé yào* 合藥). Lastly, it can mean "to shut" or "enclose."

We can, of course, read it here simply, as most commentators following Wáng Bīng have done, as a reference to the six hand and foot pairs of the twelve cardinal channels in tri-fold subdivisions of Yīn and Yáng, a reading that is suggested by other *Nèi Jīng* passages:

* * *

Commentary by Wáng Bīng 王冰

六合，謂十二經脈之合也。《靈樞經》曰：太陰陽明為一合，少陰太陽為一合，厥陰少陽為一合，手足之脈各三，則為六合也。手厥陰則心包絡脈也。

The Six Matchings are here referring to the matchings of the twelve Channel Vessels. As the Líng Shū states: "Tàiyīn and Yángmíng constitute one match. Shàoyīn and Tàiyáng constitute one match. Juéyīn and Shàoyáng constitute one match. Because there are three each of vessels of the hands and feet, there are a total of six matches. The Hand Juèyīn then is the Pericardium Network Vessel."

* * *

These gradations of Yīn and Yáng can then further be read as the progressive levels of disease penetration into the body, as laid out in the *Shāng Hán Lùn*. Such a connection is, however, not stated explicitly in the *Nèi Jīng*, and we need to be careful. Even though these six gradations of Yīn and Yáng are commonly referred to in

English as "Six Conformations," especially in the context of *Shāng Hán Lùn* -style diagnosis and treatment, it is important to note that the *Shāng Hán Lùn* does not contain either of the terms *liù jīng* 六經 (six channels) or *liù hé* 六合 (six matchings). Moreover, *Sù Wèn* 6, while explaining the six channel pairings as subdivisions of Yīn and Yáng, refers to them as three Yáng and three Yīn channels (三經), but uses the term *hé* 合 "match" only in the compound *lí hé* 離合 ("differentiating and uniting" or "separating and coming together").

Much more commonly in classical literature, the compound term *liù hé* 六合 refers to the six directions (north, south, east, west, and up and down) that enclose the universe of material reality, and therefore the totality of existence Under Heaven (see *Sù Wèn* 3 for a perfect example of this usage). This reading is suggested by a passage in the *Zhuāngzi*:

* * *

Quotation from Zhuāngzi[2]

六合之外，聖人存而不論；六合之內，聖人論而不議。。。

What is outside the Six Matchings,
the sage is present in yet does not discuss.
What is within the Six Matchings,
the sage discusses but does not dispute."

* * *

In the context of that passage, the phrase suggests a boundary, a "lid," that delineates tangible material existence, that which you can grasp intellectually and therefore discuss, from that which is beyond the realm of speech and intellectual comprehension. Based on the etymology of the character, which involves the notion of two

[2] *Zhuāngzi* 《莊子》 Chapter 2, *Qí Wù Lùn* 齊物論 (Discourse on Evening Things Out).

wings closing as a perfect match on top of things, like a two-winged door or a two-part lid that seals off a container, Dr. Brenda Hood suggests "congruence" as a possible translation for *hé* 合, which strikes me as another beautiful and quite appropriate choice. Elisabeth Rochat de la Vallée uses "six junctions" while Unschuld and Tessenow chooses "six unions," which are both also fairly close in meaning to my own choice. What is significant here is the fact that all these scholarly contemporary translators, including myself, leave the meaning of the term open to the reader's interpretation. Both Vallée and Unschuld and Tessenow do, however, follow the majority of Chinese clinical commentators in interpreting this term as referring to the six matching pairs of Yīn-Yáng channels in their discussions or choice of quoted commentaries.

Regardless of our specific word choice for translating *liù hé*, numerology is highly significant in Chinese traditional culture. It is therefore certainly not a coincidence that there are six of these pairs or matchings. Six encompasses the totality of existence as the doubling of the sacred triad of Heaven, Humanity, and Earth, or the combination of this trinity with the dynamic duality of Yīn and Yáng. The importance of the number five is well known to anybody familiar with traditional Chinese culture and medicine, but groupings in sixes are almost as frequent. Thus we have, for example, the Six *Fǔ* Organs in medicine, the Six Pitch Pipes, the Six Virtues, the Six Qì (i.e., pathological climatic factors), the hexagrams of the *Yì Jīng*, and the Six Arts. In conclusion, the expression *liù hé* most likely is a reference here to the comprehensive gridwork of vertical channels and horizontal network vessels that covers the entirety of the human body, in an intentional allusion to the concept of the Six Directions (the four cardinal directions and up and down).

Moving on, the next difficult phrase we encounter is *xī gǔ shǔ gǔ* 溪谷屬骨, which I have translated literally as "attachments of the 'ravines' and 'valleys' [of the flesh] to the bone." The "Discourse on Qì Holes" (《氣穴論》, *Sù Wèn* Chapter 58), which Wáng Bīng and most other commentators cite to explain this expression, states: "The great gatherings of the flesh are called valleys, the small gatherings of the flesh are called ravines" (肉之大會為谷，肉之小會為溪). Some commentators interpret the last two characters 屬骨 specifically as a reference to the joints as the location where bones attach to each other.

Lastly, the compound *jīng jì* 經紀 is a combination of two common compounds with very similar meanings: *jīng wěi* 經緯 "warp and woof," and *gāng jì* 綱紀 "guide rope and connecting threads" (See the discussion of the compound *gāng jì* 綱紀 in the beginning of Section One above).

* * *

Commentary by Zhāng Zhìcōng 張志聰

帝言人之臟腑形身，與天之四時陰陽外內相應，惟上古聖人，能論理人形，與天地參合。是以岐伯論天之五方、五氣、五色、五音，地之五行、五味，以應人之五體、五臟、五竅、五志也。

六合，謂十二經脈之合也。足太陽與足少陰為一合，足少陽與足厥陰為二合，足陽明與足太陰為三合，手太陽與手少陰為四合，手少陽與手厥陰為五合，手陽明與手太陰為六合者，各從其經正而相通也。

氣穴者，經氣所注之穴，有三百六十五穴，以應一歲，而各有定處，各有定名也。

谿穀者，大小之分肉，連於骨而生起也。分部者，皮之分部也。皮部中之浮絡，分三陰三陽，有順有逆，各有條理也。言天地之四時陰陽，盡有經緯紀綱，應人形之外內，皆有表有裡也。

When the Emperor speaks of the mutual inner-outer resonance between the human body with its Zàng and Fǔ Organs and the Four Seasons and Yīn and Yáng in Heaven, it is only the sages of the most ancient antiquity who were able to 'discuss and pattern the human body in accordance with deeper organizing principles,' to match it perfectly with Heaven and Earth. This is the reason why Qí Bó discusses the Five Directions, Five Qì, Five Colors, and Five Sounds in Heaven, and Five Dynamic Agents and Five Flavors on Earth, to have them resonate with the Five Body Constituents, Five Zàng Organs, Five Orifices, and Five Wills.

The "Six Matchings" refers to the matches among the Twelve Channels: The Foot Tàiyáng and Foot Shàoyīn form the first match; the Foot Shàoyáng and Foot Juéyīn form the second match; the Foot Yángmíng and Foot Tàiyīn form the third match; the Hand Tàiyáng and Hand Shàoyīn form the fourth match; the Hand Shàoyáng and Hand Juéyīn form the fifth match; and the Hand Yángmíng and Hand Tàiyīn form the sixth match. The way in which they each follow their Channel is straight and mutually connected [with their match].

The "Qì holes" are the holes that the Channel Qì pours into. There are 365 of these holes, which resonates with one year, and they each have their fixed location and their fixed name. The "ravines and valleys" are the large and small divisions in the flesh, attached to the bone and originating from there. The "spatial divisions and specific sections" are the spatial divisions and specific sections in the skin, the superficial network vessels inside the skin sections, which are divided into three Yīn and three Yáng, with some flowing along with the current and others flowing against the current, each with their own arrangement and organizing principle. When the text speaks of the Four Seasons and Yīn and Yáng in Heaven and Earth, how every single aspect of them has warp and weft, guide rope and connecting threads, and how they resonate with the outside and inside of the human body, this means that they all have an exterior and an interior aspect.

* * *

* * *

Commentary by Z'ev Rosenberg

As unfamiliar as it might seem to many clinicians, when practicing classical forms of Chinese or Asian medicine based on the Han dynasty classics, one needs to visualize internally the patterning of the human being in light of the greater forces of Heaven and Earth. One of the purposes of studying the *Sù Wèn* is to visualize and internalize this "architectural body" described by Elisabeth Hsu as upper, middle, and lower body (*sān jālo* 三焦

Triple Warmer), internal (yīn) and external (yáng) body, front and back, six hand and six foot channels, along with the 'architectural blueprints' of the Eight Extraordinary Vessels (*qí jīng bā mài* 奇經八脈) and Five Transport Point (*wǔ shū xué* 五輸穴) resonances described in the *Líng Shū* and *Nàn Jīng*. Once the physician has internalized this "clinical gaze," one views one's patient and their resonant "architecture." One sees where the flow of Qì and Blood is blocked, counter-flowing, or perturbed, and can then choose to treat to restore *yìng* 應 resonance to the patient with the heavenly and earthly Qì. In a sense, the physician is "plugging in" to an expansive present tense that references the past development of any present disorder, while also visualizing the direction in which the physician and patient would like to see health progress into the future. Using the pulse, visual, and palpation methods, one locates the disorder in the here and now and decisively resolves the pattern of disharmony.

Because Chinese medicine sees health and illness as moving, transforming states of change, its underlying principles are built to develop this awareness. Foreground (present disease patterns) and background (the patient's constitution, emotional state, the season, climate, weather, and lifestyle or dietary considerations) are always considered. With each and every patient, we are *hé* 合 joining with them as a mirror, applying clinical judgment to gently (or with intensity, depending on the situation) adjust the flow of Qì, Blood and *jīng* Essence like a river with its roots in the past and its growth into the future.

* * *

Section Seven

岐伯對曰：東方生風，風生木，木生酸，酸生肝，肝生筋，筋生心，肝主目。

其在天為玄，在人為道，在地為化。

化生五味，道生智，玄生神。

Qí Bó duì yuē: Dōng fāng shēng fēng,
fēng shēng mù, mù shēng suān,
suān shēng gān, gān shēng jīn,
jīn shēng xīn, gān zhǔ mù.

Qí zài tiān wéi xuán, zài rén wéi dào,
zài dì wéi huà.

Huà shēng wǔ wèi, dào shēng zhì,
xuán shēng shén.

Qí Bó answered: "The eastern direction engenders Wind, Wind engenders Wood, Wood engenders sourness, sourness engenders the Liver, the Liver engenders the sinews, the sinews engender the Heart, the Liver rules the eyes.

In the realm of Heaven, [the changes of Yīn and Yáng] constitute ineffable darkness; in the human realm, they constitute the Dào; in the realm of Earth, they constitute generative transformation.

Generative transformation engenders the Five Flavors; the Dào engenders wisdom; ineffable darkness engenders Shén.

With this section, Qí Bó begins his answer to the Yellow Emperor, laying out how exactly the ancients envisioned the specific resonance of the Five Dynamic Agents in Heaven, in the human body, and on Earth. In this context, it might surprise us that these five sections are not organized by the Dynamic Agents (Wood, Fire, Earth, Metal, and Water) as we might expect but by the Five Directions (east, south, center, west, and north). This detail can perhaps serve as a reminder of the importance of the cosmic body and of the role of the doctor in integrating the human body within the greater environment, which is something that can easily get lost in our contemporary model of providing healthcare.

For a discussion on the significance of the term *huà* 化, translated above as "generative transformation," as a specific type of change, and on the difference between this kind of change and the notion of *biàn* 變 (gradual alteration), see the first discussion in Section One above. Its placement in the passage above in the section on the east is significant and certainly makes contextual sense, since the east is associated with spring, with sprouting and birth and the generative energy of plants bursting through the surface of the Earth and reaching up to Heaven. Nevertheless, Lines Two and Three of this Section need to be treated with care: Given the strict parallel sentence pattern from Section Seven to Section Eleven and the grammatical difficulty in fitting these two lines smoothly into the text above, it is a reasonable assumption held by a majority of historical and contemporary commentators that Lines Two and Three are commentary or additional text from elsewhere that was inserted into the main text by an early copyist and then mistakenly incorporated as part of the source text. Following these scholars, I also include the first character of the following passage (神 *shén*) in this grouping. I have marked this reading by adding square brackets around the characters that most scholars suspect to be a later insertion, but also want to give the discerning reader the option of contemplating them as part of the text.

Whether they were originally part of the original source text, simply misplaced in this section, or come from an unrelated text, their meaning is intriguing: For comparison and additional insight on Lines Two and Three, let us look at a parallel passage from *Sù Wèn*

神在天為風，在地為木，在體為筋，在臟為肝，在色為蒼，在音為角，在聲為呼，在變動為握，在竅為目，在味為酸，在志為怒。

怒傷肝，悲勝怒；風傷筋，燥勝風；酸傷筋，辛勝酸。

Shén zài tiān wéi fēng, zài dì wéi mù, zài tǐ wéi jīn, zài zàng wéi gān, zài sè wéi cāng, zài yīn wéi jué, zài shēng wéi hū, zài biàn dòng wéi wò, zài qiào wéi mù, zài wèi wéi suān, zài zhì wéi nù.

Nù shāng gān, bēi shèng nù; fēng shāng jīn, zào shèng fēng; suān shāng jīn, xīn shèng suān.

[Shén,] in Heaven, constitutes Wind; on Earth, Wood; among the physical constituents, the Sinews; among the Zàng Organs, the Liver; among the hues, pale green; among the musical notes, jué; among the sounds [of the human voice], shouting; among the pathological movements, clenching; among the openings, the eyes; among the flavors, sourness; among the Wills, anger.

Anger injures the Liver, but grief prevails over anger. Wind injures the sinews but Parching prevails over Wind. Sourness injures the sinews, but acridity prevails over sourness.

Chapter 66, one of the later additions by Wáng Bīng in his edition of the *Sù Wèn* from 762 CE, which begins with an almost literal quotation of the introduction to the present chapter, *Sù Wèn* Chapter 5.

Quotation from Sù Wèn[1]

夫五運陰陽者，天地之道也，萬物之綱紀，變化之父母，
生殺之本始，神明之府也，可不通乎？

故物生謂之化，物極謂之變，陰陽不測謂之神，神用無方謂之聖。

夫變化之為用也，在天為玄，在人為道，
在地為化。化生五味，道生智，玄生神。

神在天為風，在地為木，在天為熱，在地為火，在天為
濕，在地為土，在天為燥，在地為金，在天為寒，在地為
水。故在天為氣，在地成形，形氣相感而化生萬物矣。

Now the Five Movements and Yīn and Yáng, these are the Dào of Heaven and Earth, the guide ropes and connecting threads of the myriad things, the father and mother of gradual alterations and generative transformations, the foundation and beginning of giving birth and taking life, and the palace of shén míng. How could you not comprehend this!

As such, the creation of things is what we refer to as 'generative transformation', while the culmination of things is referred to as 'alteration'. The unfathomable [aspect of] Yīn and Yáng is what we refer to as Shén, while the practical application of this Shén without having directions is referred to as 'sagely'.

[1] *Sù Wèn* 《素問》 Chapter 66, *Tiān Yuán Jì Dà Lùn* 天元紀大論 (Great Discourse on the Record of Heaven's Origin).

Now the practical application of alterations and transformations, in Heaven it is ineffable darkness; in the human realm it is the Dào, and on Earth it is generative transformation. Transformation engenders the Five Flavors, the Dào engenders wisdom, and ineffable darkness engenders the Shén.

Shén in Heaven is Wind, on Earth is Wood; in Heaven is Cold, on Earth is Fire; in Heaven is Dampness, on Earth is soil; in Heaven is Dryness, on Earth is Metal; in Heaven is Cold, on Earth is Water. Therefore in Heaven it is the [climatic] Qì, and on Earth it completes the Form. Form and Qì stimulate each other and transformatively engender the Myriad Things!

* * *

THIS PASSAGE FROM *SÙ WÈN* CHAPTER 66 INCLUDES ALMOST LITERALLY identical lines to our source text in *Sù Wèn* Chapter 5. While equally obscure and shrouded in "ineffable darkness," hopefully it can help to shed a tiny ray of light on these lines. We can certainly choose to explain Lines 2 and 3 of this section as an erroneous insertion by an ignorant copyist and therefore make an argument to ignore them as lines from elsewhere that do not belong in the present context. Alternatively, we can accept this challenge to grasp the meaning of one of the more difficult passages in this chapter, which is what I am going to do in the next few paragraphs.

What is the text trying to express with this statement: "In the realm of Heaven, [the changes of Yīn and Yáng] constitute ineffable darkness; in the human realm, they constitute the Dào; in the realm of Earth, they constitute generative transformation. Generative transformation engenders the Five Flavors; the Dào engenders wisdom; ineffable darkness engenders *Shén*"? Is it just a coincidence that this text is placed here at the beginning of Qí Bó's answer, or can the context of this chapter help us make sense? And if so, how do these phrases contribute to the meaning of the text before and after these two lines?

This passage occurs at a key turning point in the conversation between Qí Bó and the Yellow Emperor in this chapter. Up to here, Qí Bó's introduction has been correlating the changes of Yīn and Yáng in the macrocosm with the manifestations thereof in overlapping and sometimes not clearly differentiated microcosms: first in the seasonal changes and weather patterns in Sections One and Two (e.g., "clear Yáng is Heaven, turbid Yīn is Earth; Earth Qì rising forms clouds; Heaven Qì descending forms rain…"), and then in the nature of foods, medicinal substances, and "Fire" and their effect on the human body in Section Three, in the discussion of Qì and Flavor. Sections Four and Five then spell out the pathological effects of a disturbed equilibrium between Yīn and Yáng and between Cold and Heat on the human body, also incorporating the Five Dynamic Agents in their manifestations as the Five Emotions or "wills" (*wǔ zhì* 五志) by "transforming the Five Qì" (*huà wǔ qì* 化五氣)."

This comprehensive and sometimes presumably intentionally multi-layered monologue contains many instances where a phrase, like "double/severe Yīn must turn into Yáng; double/severe Yáng must turn into Yīn," can and probably does refer to both the macrocosmic changes and to the resulting changes in nature, in food and medicine, and in human physiology or pathology. In a seemingly abrupt change in topic, the Yellow Emperor now asks Qí Bó in Section Six for much more specific information on how the ancient sages "patterned the human body in accordance with deeper organizing principles, arrayed and differentiated the *Zàng* and *Fǔ* Organs, and laid out the Channels and Vessels in a grid of vertical stems and horizontal branches." Apparently, he wants Qí Bó to bring the lofty discourse of the first few sections down to the concrete micro-level of channel courses, locations and names of "Qì holes," attachments of flesh to bone, and circulation in the spatial divisions of the skin, to learn how these are affected by the "Four Seasons and Yīn and Yáng." For obvious reasons, Qí Bó's answer carries great weight for any student or practitioner of Chinese medicine.

And indeed, the remainder of the chapter focuses more tightly and directly on the effects of Yīn and Yáng on the human body. As such, it provides practical guidelines for diagnosis as well as treatment from different angles, but all related to the theme of this chapter, namely the manifestations of Yīn and Yáng in the human body. This discussion starts out, in Sections Seven through Eleven, with the correlations of the Five Directions (the four cardinal directions and the center) and

Five Dynamic Agents with various aspects of the human body. This is followed in Section Twelve with advice on "conforming to Yīn and Yáng" (*fǎ yīn yáng* 法陰陽), and then from Section Fourteen on for the rest of the chapter, with perhaps the most pressing question of the whole text: "How do we go about attuning these two?

Given this context, let us revisit the presumably inserted Lines Two and Three above ("In the realm of Heaven, [the changes of Yīn and Yáng] constitute ineffable darkness; in the human realm, they constitute the Dào; in the realm of Earth, they constitute generative transformation. Generative transformation engenders the Five Flavors; the Dào engenders wisdom; ineffable darkness engenders the *Shén*"). What is the vertical thread on the Heaven-Human-Earth axis that connects ineffable darkness, the Dào, and *huà*-type change, and how do these engender a second axis, of the *Shén*, wisdom, and the Five Flavors? And from a horizontal perspective, how are ineffable darkness and *Shén* related in Heaven, the Dào and wisdom in the human realm, and *huà* transformation and the Five Flavors in the realm of Earth?

In my mind, just by asking these questions, the answer, even if ultimately beyond the reach of words and rational understanding, is beginning to form. As the previous sections have clearly demonstrated over and over, Qì and Yīn-Yáng are the one semantic tool that we have at our disposal to simultaneously express the processes of change that take place at each of these levels. In my current, admittedly woefully limited and ever-developing, interpretation, these two lines can be read as a striking expression of the synthesis of three ways of looking at the universe. Starting with what we might refer to as a "Daoist" and a "Confucian" perspective, related to the realms of Heaven and Humanity, respectively, we can perhaps even add a third, clinically-oriented approach, a literally most "down-to-earth" perspective, from which we might be able to relate these other levels of insight to the theories and practices of Chinese medicine. Far too often, the perfectly round peg of the Yellow Emperor's Inner Classic or of Chinese medicine as a whole is forced into the square hole of either Daoist or Confucian philosophical approaches, resulting in the unfortunate loss of its integrity, internal coherence, and, perhaps most importantly, clinical efficacy.

When reading the text in this fashion, what the passage is expressing here is the need to view the world, our human role in it, and the concrete application of this understanding in clinical action, from all three angles: To start from the bottom (and perhaps easiest because most tangible aspect) up, the "Five Flavors" in the realm of Earth concern life and health on the most basic level, as the directly visible effect of foods and medicinal substances on the human body. We are what we eat, after all. As such, too much of any one food is bound to disturb the sensitive equilibrium in the body, especially if we consume medicinally active substances with "thick" Flavors and Qì. It is no coincidence that Section Three on the Flavors above contains the stern warnings that "the Qì of Strong Fire weakens" and that "Strong Fire eats Qì…[and] scatters Qì." The effects of introducing an excess of Yīn or Yáng into the body by ingesting excessively cold or hot foods are, after all, an easily graspable example of how excess Yīn or Yáng manifest in the body. Here we are of course not talking about cold and hot foods in terms of their temperature but in terms of their nature and effect on the body. But we should perhaps also understand the "Five Flavors" in a larger sense, namely as the product of "what *huà* transformation engenders" (化生五味). As such, Earth is the realm where the "Form" *xíng* 形 is completed *chéng* 成. This is the visible, tangible, literally taste-able aspect of Qì in the universe, easily experienced by oral ingestion. And this creative process is precisely what that difficult term *huà* 化 refers to. Translated into the context of clinical work, for most doctors this should be the easiest level at which to diagnose and then treat dis-equilibrium in the human body. And it seems to me that this is also the level at which modern biomedicine is most comfortable practicing. In conclusion then, the passage "In the realm of Earth, [the changes of Yīn and Yáng] constitute generative transformation. Generative transformation engenders the Five Flavors," thus may be read in this way: The dynamic, generative, ceaseless interplay of Yīn and Yáng, in the realm of Earth, manifests as *huà*-type change, or in other words sudden, abrupt, substantive change, specifically from non-being into being, resulting in the creation and destruction, living and dying, of the material world. Through this change, Yīn and Yáng produce the Myriad Things, which are here referred to specifically as the "Five Flavors" to emphasize not only their association with the Five Dynamic Agents but also their role in affecting, positively or negatively, the human body when they are ingested as food. As such they represent Qì materialized into Form, which through its correlation with the Five Dynamic Agents affects the state of the Qì of the Five *Zàng* Organs in the body.

Moving on from the realm of Earth to the two upper levels, namely the realms of Humanity and Heaven, the text tells us: "In the realm of Heaven, [the changes of Yīn and Yáng] constitute ineffable darkness; in the human realm, they constitute the Dào"... and "the Dào engenders wisdom, ineffable darkness engenders *Shén*." The key terms here are Dào 道 and "wisdom" (*zhì* 智), as the terms associated with Humanity, and "ineffable darkness" (*xuán* 玄) and *Shén* 神 in the realm of Heaven, which run parallel with "generative transformation" and the Five Flavors in the realm of Earth. As we have already encountered elsewhere in this text, the realm of Heaven is characterized by being unfathomable, unknowable, beyond the limit of ordinary human comprehension, and therefore "dark." In some versions of this passage, the character *xuán* 玄 is actually replaced by its close relative *yuán* 元, "primordial," which looks and sounds quite similar and is therefore an easy change to make for a copyist or scribe who is writing down an oral transmission. While these two words don't seem related in modern English, readers familiar with Chinese cosmology know the closeness in meaning between ineffable darkness and the primordial as two key concepts to describe the origin of creation before differentiation and manifestation in Form in the progression from none to one to two to five to the "Myriad Things." To understand how this primordial darkness then engenders *Shén*, it might help to remember the definition of *Shén* that I quoted in the very first section of this text in the explanation of the compound *shén míng* "spirit brightness": "What is immeasurable/unfathomable in Yīn and Yáng is called *Shén*." In other words, the interactions of Yīn and Yáng in Heaven are unknowable and mysterious. In contrast, the realm of Humanity is characterized by Dào, by a path, or in other words a succession of changes that can be perceived, followed, expressed, explained, and comprehended. And once we understand this cosmic Dào, in the sense of the Way of Change through the interaction of Yīn and Yáng in the manifest world, we have obtained "wisdom" as the ability to grasp, respond to, and align ourselves with these changes. This is, after all, the key to nurturing life in the way of the ancient sages and the essence of a successful human existence.

* * *

Commentary by Zhāng Zhìcōng 張志聰

其在人為道，道者，陰陽五行不易之理也。道生智，智者，五臟之神志魂魄。因思慮而處物。是以人之五臟，生五神，化五志也。

Concerning the statement, "in the human realm, [the changes of Yīn and Yáng] constitute the Dào," the Dào is the immutable organizing principle of Yīn and Yáng and the Five Dynamic Agents. This Dào engenders wisdom. And concerning this wisdom, it is the Shén, Wills, and hún and pò souls of the Five Zàng Organs that manage things because of rumination and discernment, and therefore it is the Five Zàng Organs in humans that engender the Five Shèn and generatively transform the Five Wills.

* * *

According to Zhāng, the Dào, as the principle according to which Yīn and Yáng and the Five Dynamic Agents operate, engenders wisdom in humans because it gives us the ability to "manage things." This correct engagement with our external environment takes place through our *Shén*, emotions, and *hún* and *pò* souls, as a consequence of the active application of thought and discernment. This reminds me of the famous progression of knowledge laid out in the *Dà Xué* 《大學》 (Great Learning) where the ruler's ability to create and maintain order in the state is rooted in a succession of skills that zoom in progressively from his ability to make his family harmonious to cultivating his person to straightening out the heart to making the intention sincere to perfecting knowing/wisdom to investigating things. Whether for the healer or the ruler, the careful and conscious engagement with the "myriad things," or in other words with the external environment from food to clothing to sexual intercourse to political, medical, and all other activities in accordance with the fluctuations of Yīn and Yáng and the progression of the Five Dynamic Agents is the outward expression of this wisdom. And this wisdom in turn can be defined as the ability to live in alignment with the Dào, to go along with the current instead of striving to move against it.

Returning to *Sù Wèn* Chapter 5 and the list of resonances associated with the East as the first of the Five Directions, the remainder of this Section is much more straightforward and should be familiar to any reader trained in the theoretical foundations of Chinese medicine, with the exception of two terms that require an explanation: My translation of *biàn dòng* 變動 as "pathological movement" tries to capture the intended meaning of this verbal phrase here and in the following four sections. To get a better sense of this compound term, which literally means "transformation movements," in the present context, let us look at each of the Five-Agent associations: Liver-Wood-east with clenching, Heart-Fire-south with mourning, Spleen-Earth-center with dry heaving, Lung-Metal-west with coughing, and Kidney-Water-north with trembling. With the exception of the Heart, the terms describe abnormal physical movements that are the result of pathological changes related to the organ in question. As such, they offer a diagnostic clue that allows the attentive physician to detect a problem with one of these five aspects before it manifests in serious illness. In other words, the compound *biàn dòng* 變動 describes a change 變 in the physical condition of the body that manifests in a movement 動. For a discussion on the movement associated with the Heart, see my explanation on page 177 below on yōu 憂 (mourning) in Section Eight on south-Fire-Heart. In addition and related to this character, it should be noted that the state of mind associated with the Lung here, grief (*bēi* 悲), is different from the term used in the section on the Lung itself, namely *yōu* 憂 (mourning).

To give just one example of the standard way in which this Section on the east and the following four Sections on the south, center, west, and north are usually interpreted, here is the commentary by Mǎ Shì. Especially the last two paragraphs shed light on how we should read this part of the Great Discourse.

* * *

Commentary by Mǎ Shì 馬蒔

東方主春，陽氣上升，故東方生風。風鼓則木榮，故風生木。木之性曲直作酸，故木生酸。人身之肝屬木，木性屬酸，故酸生肝。諸筋者皆屬於肝，故肝生筋。木主生火，故筋生心。目者肝之竅，故肝主目。

又嘗即天地人而統言之，不過一理焉耳。其在天也為玄，玄者冥漠之稱；其在人也為道，道者共由之理；其在地也為化，化者造物之能。惟地有是化，則品物形而五味生；惟人有是道，則大道彰而明智生；惟天有是玄，則玄功若而至神生。此可見三才惟一理也。

又嘗即前所言者而極推之，其在天五氣為風，在地五行為木，在人五體為筋，在五臟為肝，在五色為蒼。。。名雖萬殊，理無二。致皆屬之於木而已。

然本臟之太過者，反有所傷，而惟本臟之所不勝者，為能制之也。故在志為怒，怒太過則傷肝，惟肺金主悲，為能勝怒;在天為風，風氣通於肝則傷筋，惟西方燥金為能勝風；在味為酸，酸太過則傷筋，惟西方味辛，為能勝酸。此皆金能剋木，故制其所勝者如此。

The eastern direction is in charge of spring and Yáng Qì rising; therefore the eastern direction engenders Wind. Wind billowing makes trees thrive; therefore Wind engenders Wood. The nature of Wood is bending and straightening and it produces sourness; therefore Wood engenders sourness. In the human body, the Liver is associated with Wood, and the nature of Wood is associated with sourness; therefore sourness engenders the Liver. All the various sinews are associated with the Liver; therefore the Liver engenders the sinews. Wood is in charge of engendering Fire;

therefore the sinews engender the Heart. The eyes are the orifices of the Liver; therefore the Liver is in charge of the eyes.

Now, speaking from the perspective of integrating Heaven, Earth, and Humanity, they all operate by a single guiding principle, and that is all! In the realm of Heaven, this [principle] is ineffable darkness. Ineffable darkness is the designation for that which is obscure and abstruse. In the realm of Humanity, this [principle] is the Dào. The Dào is the principle of the shared cause. In the realm of Earth, this [principle] is generative transformation. Generative transformation is the capacity to construct things. It is only when in the realm of Earth this generative transformation exists that articles and things take Form and the Five Flavors are engendered. It is only when in the realm of Humanity this Dào exists that the Great Dào is resplendent and illuminated wisdom is engendered. And it is only when in the realm of Heaven this ineffable darkness exists that the ineffable darkness achieves concordance and the ultimate Shén is engendered. From this we can see how the Three Powers operate under a single guiding principle.

Now, if we extend what has been said above to its furthest limit, in Heaven among the Five [climatic] Qì, it constitutes Wind; on Earth among the Five Dynamic Agents it constitutes Wood; in humans among the five physical constituents it is the sinews; among the Five Zàng Organs it is the Liver; among the Five Hues it is pale green;....Even though there are a myriad differences in the names, the guiding principle is only one, namely that they are all associate¬d with Wood and that is all.

This being so, when the Zàng Organ discussed here is in a state of great excess and we see injury instead [of healthy physiology], only that aspect that this Zàng Organ does not prevail over is able to control it. As such, among the Wills, [east/Wood] constitutes anger, and when anger is greatly excessive, it injures the Liver. Now, it is only Lung Metal, being in charge of grief, that is able to prevail over anger. In Heaven, [east/Wood] constitutes Wind, and when Wind Qì penetrates to the Liver, it injures the sinews. It is only Dryness Metal of the western direction that is able to prevail over Wind. Among the Flavors, [east/Wood] constitutes sourness, and when sourness is greatly excessive, it injures the sinews. It is only the acrid flavor of the western direction that is able to prevail over sourness. All of these examples are cases of Metal being able to subdue Wood and thereby controlling that which it prevails over.

Section Eight

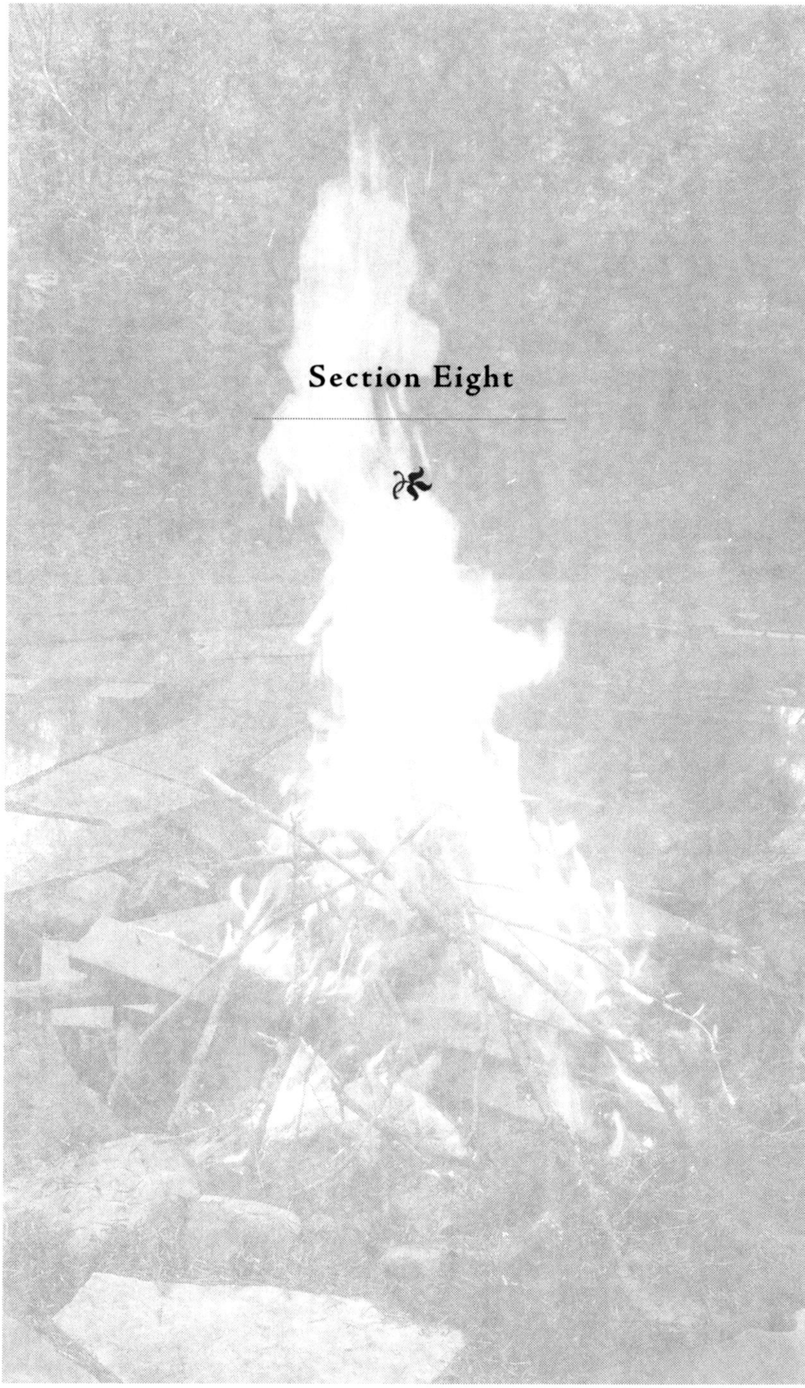

南方生熱，熱生火，火生苦，苦生心，心生血，血生脾，心主舌。
其在天為熱，在地為火，在體為脈，在臟為心，在色為赤，在音為徵，
在聲為笑，在變動為憂，在竅為舌，在味為苦，在志為喜。

Nán fāng shēng rè, rè shēng huǒ, huǒ shēng kǔ, kǔ shēng xīn, xīn shēng xuè, xuè shēng pí, xīn zhǔ shé.

Qí zài tiān wéi rè, zài dì wéi huǒ, zài tǐ wéi mài, zài zàng wéi xīn, zài sè wéi chì, zài yīn wéi zhēng, zài shēng wéi xiào, zài biàn dòng wéi yōu, zài qiào wéi shé, zài wèi wéi kǔ, zài zhì wéi xǐ.

The southern direction engenders Heat, Heat engenders Fire, Fire engenders bitterness, bitterness engenders the Heart, the Heart engenders Blood, Blood engenders the Spleen, the Heart rules the tongue.

In Heaven, it constitutes Heat; on Earth, Fire; among the physical constituents, the Vessels; among the Zàng Organs, the Heart; among the hues, red; among the musical notes, zhǐ; among the sounds [of the human voice], laughter; among the pathological movements, mourning; among the openings, the tongue; among the flavors, bitterness; among the Wills, happiness.

THIS SECTION PROVIDES A LIST OF PROPERTIES, ACTIONS, AND aspects of the body associated with south, the Heart, and Fire that does not offer a lot of surprises to any reader familiar with basic Chinese medicine theory. The one detail that stands out and deserves a bit of attention is the emotion or "Will": In line with standard medical literature from this period, the Heart is associated with happiness (*xǐ* 喜) among the "Five Wills." In light of this, the presence of the term *yōu* 憂 "mourning" here is a bit surprising as a description of the pathological movement that indicates an unhealthy state of the constellation south-Heat-Fire-Heart. Commentators have explained it in different ways. It is the same character that is used in Section Ten below to refer to the emotion or "will" associated with the Lung. In an attempt to express the more active dimension here and reflect its textual context as a "movement" or "stirring" (*dòng* 動), one could choose to read it here as "fretting" instead. Alternatively, we could recall that the Heart stores the *Shén*, and when there is an excess of *Shén*, we see laughing, but when there is not enough *Shén*, we see its opposite, namely mourning, in the sense of a melancholy deadness or absence of spirit, a quality that we usually associate more with the Lung. This is how Zhāng Jièbīn explains the presence of "mourning" here as the pathological movement of the Heart: "The Heart stores the *Shén*, and an excess of *Shén* results in laughter, while an insufficiency of *Shén* results in mourning." We can also follow Zhāng Zhìcōng's lead and emphasize the close connection between the Heart and the Lung through Qì, as a result of which an imbalance in the Heart easily results in a manifestation of the emotional state associated with the Lung.

Before moving on to the next section, the evaluation of happiness in Chinese medicine deserves a brief discussion. Especially the United States can appear to an outsider like a hyper-positive culture of continually smiling faces where well-meaning strangers routinely and politely inquire how you are doing and respond with surprise, confusion, or consternation when they receive an honest answer that is anything less than an exuberant "Fantastic!" Abundant recent research in fields like positive psychology emphasizes the health benefits of a happy attitude towards life. Even authoritative sources like the Harvard School of

喜傷心，恐勝喜；熱傷氣，寒勝熱；苦傷氣，鹹勝苦。

Xǐ shāng xīn, kǒng shèng xǐ;
rè shāng qì, hán shèng rè;
kǔ shāng qì, xián shèng kǔ.

Happiness injures the Heart,
but fear prevails over happiness.
Heat injures the Qì,
but Cold prevails over Heat.
Bitterness injures the Qì but
saltiness prevails over bitterness.

Public Health propose that a "sunny outlook" can positively affect our susceptibility to colds, heart disease, hypertension, diabetes, and premature aging.[1] In light of such studies, we may not agree with the statement here that happiness, as the emotion associated with the Heart, is one of the Five Emotions that can be the cause of pathology. But that is precisely what the *Nèi Jīng* emphasizes over and over. It is therefore important not to alter the source text by translating 喜 xǐ as "excessive happiness" or "overexcitement" or even "agitation," as many contemporary renditions of this theory do in English. How we end up interpreting this line clinically is up to each of us individually, but for the purpose of a literal translation it is essential that "happiness" is presented in exactly the same terms as the other four emotions: anger, ruminating, mourning, and fear.

Given our potential discomfort with the statement above that "happiness injures the Heart," it is worth taking a closer look at the Chinese term for "happiness," *xǐ* 喜. In terms of its etymology, the character is a combination of drum 鼓 with mouth 口, and therefore presumably expresses the happiness experienced during festivals like weddings, with lots of drumming and singing and perhaps some wild drinking and dancing. This is also the character that, in the doubled-up version of 喜喜 is ubiquitously painted on everything from vases to match boxes, jewelry, and wedding announcements, and hung upside down around the home of married couples.

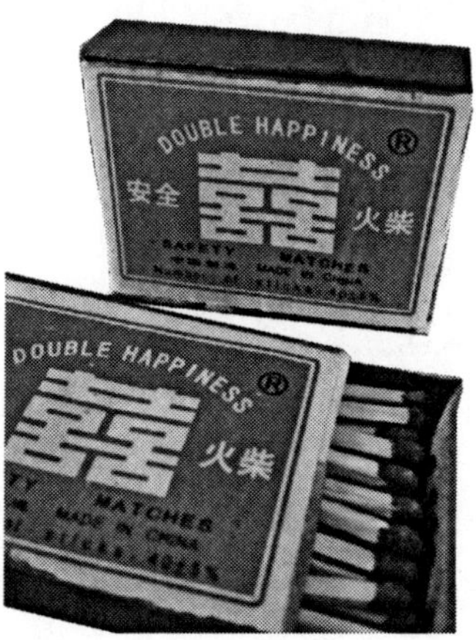

It is thus definitely not a word with a negative connotation like "agitation," but rather a positive term, just like the English notion of happiness. My own word choice is similar to Elisabeth Rochat de la Vallée's translation as "elation" and Unschuld and Tessenow's as "joy" in avoiding a term with inherently negative connotations in English.

[1] www.hsph.harvard.edu/news/magazine/happiness-stress-heart-disease, 3/16/2018.

It is helpful to contrast the precise meaning of *xǐ* 喜 with another Chinese character, *lè* 樂, which it is often combined with in more contemporary literature. The character for *lè* 樂 is also related to music, and even has the meaning "music" in the alternate pronunciation *yuè*, but depicts a very different kind of instrument: a wooden rack with dangling objects. As such it is not a casual hand drum used in rowdy and ecstatic village celebrations but an elaborate assemblage, whether with jade pieces, stones, or even bronze bells, that is played in serious and refined rituals such as ceremonies at court to produce vibrations that harmonize the human realm of the ritual participants with Heaven. In contrast to the solemn Yīn quality of *lè* 樂, the character 喜 reflects the uplifting, outgoing Yáng quality of a jovial, celebratory kind of happiness.[2]

As mentioned elsewhere throughout this book and in numerous passages in the Chinese philosophical and medical classics, happiness is in classical Chinese culture seen as one of the Five Emotions that affect the heart and *Shén*. The Heart is the seat of the *Shén* and thus carries the essential function of holding and housing the *Shén,* preventing it from floating astray or scattering, as it is likely to do when perturbed by any of the emotions. Happiness creates movement, frees up blockage, shakes things up, and literally "lifts the spirit." This freeing quality is beneficial in moderation but, in the Chinese view, can endanger the Heart's tenuous hold over the *Shén*. Like all the other emotions, happiness is an internal response to an external stimulus that upsets the equilibrium and causes judgment of things or events as "good" versus "bad" or "right" versus "wrong." This human tendency to ascribe value then prevents us from responding with equanimity and clarity, aligning ourselves with the Dào and surrendering to the flow of the current. As a result of human effort and striving, our lives are cut short and we are unable to live out our Heavenly allotted lifespan in the manner of the ancient sages. As the Daoist philosopher *Zhuāngzi* loves to point out, human knowledge is as limited as the perspective of a frog in a well or a dreaming butterfly.

[2] For more information on these two kinds of joy in Chinese, see Sandra Hill's blog post on "Joy": www.monkeypress.net/blog/joy#more-443.

* * *

Quotation from Zhuāngzi[3]

夔憐蚿，蚿憐蛇，蛇憐風。。。

夔謂蚿曰：「吾以一足跉踔而行，予無如矣。今子之使萬足，獨奈何？」蚿曰：「不然。子不見夫唾者乎？噴則大者如珠，小者如霧，雜而下者不可勝數也。今予動吾天機，而不知其所以然。」

蚿謂蛇曰：「吾以眾足行，而不及子之無足，何也？」蛇曰：「夫天機之所動，何可易邪？吾安用足哉！」

蛇謂風曰：「予動吾脊脅而行，則有似也。今子蓬蓬然起於北海，蓬蓬然入於南海，而似無有，何也？」風曰：「然。予蓬蓬然起於北海而入於南海也，然而指我則勝我，䲡我亦勝我。雖然，夫折大木，蜚大屋者，唯我能也，故以眾小不勝為大勝也。為大勝者，唯聖人能之。」

The one-footed kuí monster envies the millipede, the millipede envies the wind...

The kuí monster said to the millipede: "While I move forward by laboriously hopping around on one foot, you are not like that at all! Now how on earth do you manage employing ten thousand feet?" The millipede responded: "It is not like that. Have you never seen a person spit? When they spurt it out, the big drops like pearls and the small drops like mist all mixed together, they fall down in uncountable numbers. Now I [simply] move my heavenly mechanism and do not know the means by which it is like this."

The millipede said to the snake: "I move forward by means of my multitude of feet and yet I do not reach your ability to move without feet. How can that be?" The snake replied: "This being a movement by means of the heavenly mechanism, how could I change this? How could I possibly use feet!"

[3] *Zhuāngzi* 《莊子》 Chapter 17, *Qiū Shuǐ* 秋水 (Autumn Floods).

The snake said to the wind: "I move forward by activating my spine and rib-sides and therefore there is an appearance [of having feet]. Now you, on the other hand, with a huff and puff rise up from the Northern Sea, and with a huff and a puff enter the Southern Sea. And yet you appear to not even have a presence. How can that be?" The wind answered: "This is correct. As for my rising from the Northern Sea and entering the Southern Sea with a single huff and a puff, it is like this and yet, anybody can point a mere finger at me and overcome me, anybody can crawl around on me and overcome me. And yet, I am the only one who has the ability to break great trees and make great houses fly off. Therefore I use the multitude of small defeats to make one great victory. As for what a great victory is, only the sage is capable to doing that."

* * *

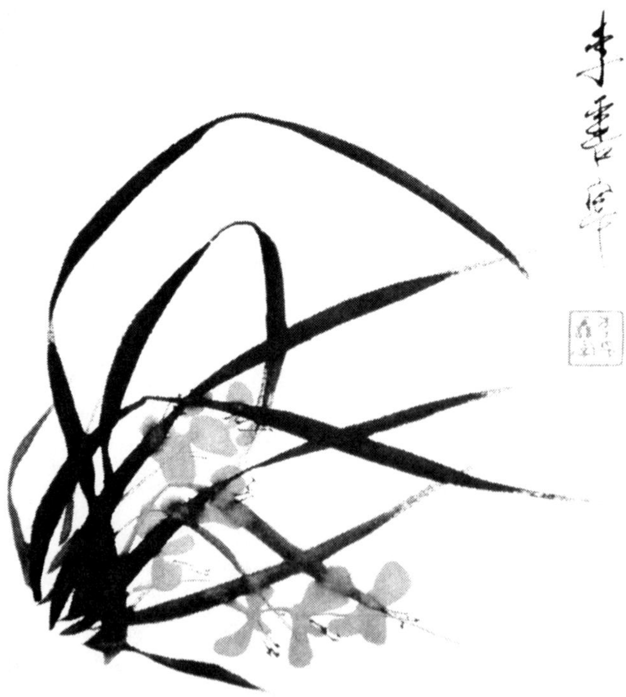

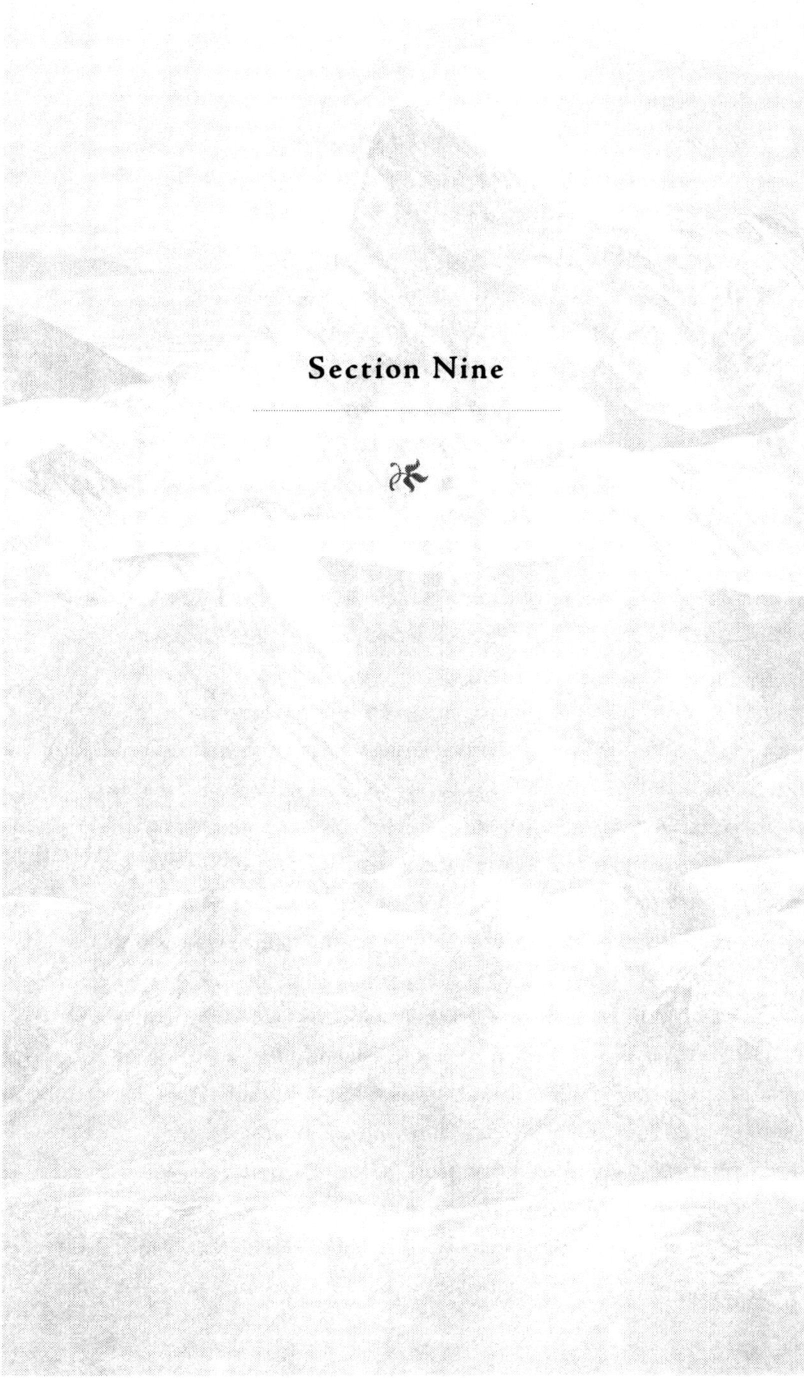

Section Nine

中央生濕，濕生土，土生甘，甘生脾，脾生肉，肉生肺，脾主口。

其在天為濕，在地為土，在體為肉，在臟為脾，在色為黃，在音為宮，

在聲為歌，在變動為噦，在竅為口，在味為甘，在志為思。

Zhōng yāng shēng shī, shī shēng tǔ,
tǔ shēng gān, gān shēng pí, pí shēng ròu,
ròu shēng fèi, pí zhǔ kǒu.

Qí zài tiān wéi shī, zài dì wéi tǔ,
zài tǐ wéi ròu, zài zàng wéi pí,
zài sè wéi huáng, zài yīn wéi gōng,
zài shēng wéi gē, zài biàn dòng wéi yuě,
zài qiào wéi kǒu, zài wèi wéi gān,
zài zhì wéi sī.

The central core engenders Dampness, Dampness engenders Earth, Earth engenders sweetness, sweetness engenders the Spleen, the Spleen engenders the flesh, the flesh engenders the Lung, the Spleen rules the mouth.

In Heaven, it constitutes Dampness; on Earth, earth; among the physical constituents, the flesh; among the Zàng Organs, the Spleen; among the hues, yellow; among the musical notes, gōng; among the sounds [of the human voice], singing; among the pathological movements, dry heaving; among the openings, the mouth; among the Flavors, sweetness; among the Wills, ruminating.

THIS SECTION DOES NOT PRESENT ANY SURPRISES OR SERIOUS textual problems. Regarding the pathological movement associated with the center-Earth-Spleen-Stomach, I follow most commentators in reading the character *yuě* 噦 literally as dry retching, or vomiting without result. Zhāng Zhìcōng explains this phenomenon as the pathological countercurrent flow of Qì in the space of the Spleen, which is located between the Lung and Stomach:

* * *

Commentary by Zhāng Zhìcōng 張志聰

氣逆於肺胃之間，則為噦。胃之上，肺之下，脾之分也。故脾氣變動則為噦。

Qì moving countercurrent in the space between the Lung and the Stomach results in dry retching. Above the Stomach and below the Lung, this is the division of the Spleen. As such, the pathological movement of Spleen Qì is dry retching.

* * *

OTHER POSSIBLE TRANSLATIONS ARE "BELCHING" OR "HICCUP."[1] IN *Líng Shū* 靈樞 Chapter 28, Qí Bó explains this specific pathology to the Yellow Emperor by stating that it is due to grain entering the Stomach, and Stomach Qì then pouring upward into the Lung. Because Cold Qì and new grain Qì have entered the Stomach together, they disorder the normal flow of Qì by combining right Qì with evil Qì. Qí Bó there recommends treatment for this condition by supplementing Hand Tàiyīn and draining Foot Shàoyīn. Unless it is a scribal error, for which I have not found a convincing argument, it is unlikely to mean belching here because the specific term for that pathology, *yī* 噫, is explained separately further down in that chapter as being due to Cold Qì entering the Stomach and scattering up and down in countercurrent Reversal.

[1] Rochat de la Vallée, 35, and Unschuld and Tessenow, 108.

思傷脾，怒勝思；濕傷肉，風勝濕；

甘傷肉，酸勝甘。

Sī shāng pí, nù shèng sī;
shī shāng ròu, fēng shèng shī;
gān shāng ròu, suān shèng gān.

Ruminating injures the Spleen
but anger prevails over ruminating.
Dampness injures the flesh
but Wind prevails over Dampness.
Sweetness injures the flesh
but sourness prevails over sweetness.

The emotion or "Will" (*zhì*) routinely associated with the Spleen-Stomach in classical Chinese medicine is 思 *sī*, which I have chosen to translate somewhat tongue-in-cheek as "ruminating." As you may know, the rumen is a part of the stomach in ruminant animals where food is broken down for digestion. And "to ruminate" means literally to repeatedly and slowly chew half-digested food particles known as "cud," or figuratively to think about something repeatedly and obsessively, rolling it around in your mind, unable to let it go. This is exactly what the Chinese term *sī* 思 expresses in its association with Earth among the Five Agents and the Spleen among the Five *Zàng* Organs. In other contexts, *sī* 思 means not only simply "to think," but also "to long for," or "to reflect on." Unschuld and Tessenow's translation as "pensiveness" may be another good choice in the present context. In my eyes, though, the literal etymological connection of the English verb "to ruminate" with the stomach makes this term the perfect fit here.

In the list of the emotions in the second line of Section Five (see page 121), the Five Wills are presented as *xǐ nù bēi yōu kǒng* 喜怒悲憂恐 "happiness, anger, grief, mourning, and fear," which is slightly different from the terms used here. Most commentators agree that the discrepancy is due to a mistake or inconsistency there, and that *bēi* 悲 "grief" should be replaced with *sī* 思 "ruminating" there. The associations of happiness with the Heart, anger with the Liver, and fear with the Kidney are clear and consistent from one text or passage to the next both within the *Nèi Jīng* corpus and in other medical literature. According to the text here and elsewhere, the "Will" associated with the Spleen is "ruminating" *sī* 思, while "mourning" (*yōu* 憂) or "grief" (*bēi* 悲), are the closely related terms associated with the Lung. Here it is significant that *bēi* 悲 is also the character used in Section Seven, above to refer to the emotion of the Lung as the one that can overcome the anger of the Liver, and that *yōu* 憂 "mourning" is mentioned as the pathological movement associated with south-Fire-Heart, which we have seen can be explained through its connection to the Lung. Regardless of the specific terms used, the emotion associated with Spleen-Earth is one of thinking, of "stewing" on things instead of letting them go, or in my choice of metaphor, of chewing them over repeatedly in the same way that ruminant animals chew their cud. While this activity in its literal sense may help a goat digest old Christmas trees, the *Nèi Jīng* here provides a helpful reminder that its mental equivalent does have negative consequences for human stomachs, in the same way that anger injures the liver and happiness injures the heart.

Lastly, this Section follows the same structure as the previous two sections on the eastern and southern direction in making some use of the shēng 生 (engendering) and kè 剋 (restraint) cycles among the Five Dynamic Agents: Thus, the flesh, associated with the Spleen and center, engenders the lung. Following the *kè* cycle in the third sentence, damage to the Spleen and flesh as the result of ruminating, dampness, and sweetness can be prevented or counteracted by the involvement of anger, wind, and sourness, all of which are associated with Liver-Wood in the east, which restrains Spleen-Earth in the center. The text thus shows how these five-fold resonances can be applied in diagnosis and treatment at the level of the emotions, climatic factors, and flavors.

Section Ten

西方生燥，燥生金，金生辛，辛生肺，肺生皮毛，皮毛生腎，肺主鼻。
其在天為燥，在地為金，在體為皮毛，在臟為肺，在色為白，在音為商，
在聲為哭，在變動為咳，在竅為鼻，在味為辛，在志為憂。

Xī fāng shēng zào, zào shēng jīn,
jīn shēng xīn, xīn shēng fèi, fèi shēng
pí máo, pí máo shēng shèn, fèi zhǔ bí.

Qí zài tiān wéi zào, zài dì wéi jīn,
zài tǐ wéi pí máo, zài zàng wéi fèi,
zài sè wéi bái, zài yīn wéi shāng,
zài shēng wéi kū, zài biàn dòng wéi ké,
zài qiào wéi bí, zài wèi wéi xīn,
zài zhì wéi yōu.

The western direction engenders
Parching, Parching engenders Metal,
Metal engenders acridity,
acridity engenders the Lung,
the Lung engenders the skin
and body hair, the skin and
body hair engender the Kidney,
the Lung rules the nose.

In Heaven, it constitutes Parching;
on Earth, Metal; among the physical
constituents, the skin and body hair;
among the Zàng Organs, the Lung;
among the hues, white;
among the musical notes, shāng;
among the sounds [of the human voice],
crying; among the pathological
movements, coughing;
among the openings, the nose;
among the Flavors, acridity;
among the Wills, mourning.

憂傷肺，喜勝憂；熱傷皮毛，寒勝熱；
辛傷皮毛，苦勝辛。

Yōu shāng fèi, xǐ shèng yōu;
rè shāng pí máo, hán shèng rè;
xīn shāng pí máo, kǔ shèng xīn.

Mourning injures the Lung,
but happiness prevails over mourning.
Heat (Parching?) injures the
skin and body hair,
but Cold prevails over
Heat(Parching?).
Acridity injures the
skin and body hair,
but bitterness prevails over acridity.

Like the previous sections, the list here repeats standard Chinese medicine theory, with just one notable exception in Line Three: *rè shāng pí máo* 熱傷皮毛 "Heat injures the skin and body hair." What are we to make of the fact that even though the climatic factor associated with the western direction and Lung-Metal has been confirmed as Parching (*zào* 燥) in the last sentence of this Section we find Heat (*rè* 熱) instead, the climatic factor that is normally associated with Fire? Admittedly the meaning of these two characters is closely related since the Chinese for "parching" makes it clear that it is a specific type of dryness that is related to heat, different from the cracked skin that one might experience as the result of exposure to cold, for example. Bear with me as this difference will become important below. There are several ways to explain the presence of Heat here in the last line: Most commentators follow the Sòng editorial team under Lín Yì 林億 and read *rè* 熱 "Heat" here as a textual error that should simply be replaced with *zào* 燥 "Parching." Given the fact that both share the fire radical and look somewhat similar, this is a reasonable proposition. Perhaps the strongest argument in support of this reading is the fact that a parallel passage in the *Tài Sù* 太素 version of the text does have *zào* 燥 here. To draw the reader's attention to this issue, I have therefore added the word "Parching" with a question mark in parentheses after "Heat."

Other commentators simply ignore the difference between the two terms, which admittedly is minor, and treat them as equivalents. Apparently following this strategy, Wáng Bīng's explanation here certainly makes good sense:

* * *

Commentary by Wáng Bīng 王冰

熱從火生，能耗津液，故傷皮毛。寒勝熱，陰制陽也。

Heat is engendered from Fire and is able to consume the fluids. Therefore it injures the skin and body hair. Cold prevailing over heat is a case of Yīn prevailing over Yáng.

* * *

In a slightly different but elegant twist, Mǎ Shì points out that Heat is simply the excess of Parching. As a result, his concluding remarks that all the situations in the last sentence of this Section are instances of Fire restraining Metal are thus strictly speaking incorrect, since in the case of the climatic factor we have Water (Cold) restraining Fire (Heat), which in turn restrains Metal (Parching), but is here simply explained as an excess of Parching. Thus he ignores the mentioning of Cold in the case of the climatic factor, which directly contradicts his conclusion. All that being said, one could of course argue from a clinical perspective that it makes more clinical sense to treat the effect of Parching (which is, after all, related etymologically to Fire and thereby to Heat) on the skin and body hair with Cold rather than with Heat. This apparent inconsistency in the text here might thus be an example of a passage where clinical meaning overrides strict Five Agents resonances.

Commentary by Mǎ Shì 馬蒔

然本臟之太過者，反有所傷，而惟本臟之所不勝者，為能勝之也。故在志為憂，憂之過者則傷肺，惟心火之喜，為能勝憂。在天為燥，燥之過者則熱，熱傷皮毛，惟北方之寒，為能勝熱。在味為辛，辛之過者，則傷皮毛，惟火味之苦，為能勝辛。此皆火能剋金，故制其所勝者如此。

A state of great excess in this Zàng Organ (i.e., the Lung) will on the contrary cause injury, and only that [Organ, Will, Climatic Factor, or Flavor] that the Lung does not prevail over is able to prevail over it instead. As such, [Lung-Metal] among the Wills constitutes mourning, an excess of mourning results in injury to the Lung, and it is only the happiness of Heart-Fire that is able to prevail over mourning. [Among the climatic factors] in Heaven, it is Parching, and the excess of Parching results in Heat. Heat injures the skin and body hair, and it is only the Cold of the northern direction that is able to prevail over Heat. Among the flavors, it constitutes acridity, and an excess of acridity results in injury to the skin and body hair. It is only the bitterness of the Fire flavor that is able to prevail over acridity. All of these instances are cases where Fire is able to restrain Metal, and demonstrate how it controls that which it prevails over.

Section Eleven

北方生寒，寒生水，水生鹹，鹹生腎，腎生骨髓，髓生肝，腎主耳。
其在天為寒，在地為水，在體為骨，在臟為腎，在色為黑，在音為羽，
在聲為呻，在變動為栗，在竅為耳，在味為鹹，在志為恐。

Běi fāng shēng hán, hán shēng shuǐ,
shuǐ shēng xián, xián shēng shèn,
shèn shēng gǔ suǐ, suǐ shēng gān, shèn zhǔ ěr.

Qí zài tiān wéi hán, zài dì wéi shuǐ,
zài tǐ wéi gǔ, zài zàng wéi shèn,
zài sè wéi hēi, zài yīn wéi yǔ,
zài shēng wéi shēn, zài biàn dòng wéi lì,
zài qiào wéi ěr, zài wèi wéi xián,
zài zhì wéi kǒng.

The northern direction engenders Cold, Cold engenders Water, Water engenders saltiness, saltiness engenders the Kidney, the Kidney engenders the bones and marrow, the marrow engenders the Liver, the Kidney rules the ears.

In Heaven, it constitutes Cold; on Earth, Water; among the physical constituents, the bones; among the Zàng Organs, the Kidney; among the hues, black; among the musical notes, yǔ; among the sounds [of the human voice], moaning; among the pathological movements, trembling; among the openings, the ears; among the Flavors, saltiness; among the Wills, fear.

恐傷腎，思勝恐；寒傷血，燥勝寒；鹹傷血，甘勝鹹。

Kǒng shāng shèn, sī shèng kǒng;
hán shāng xuè, zào shèng hán;
xián shāng xuè, gān shèng xián.

Fear injures the Kidney,
but ruminating prevails over fear.
Cold injures the Blood (bones?),
but Parching (Dampness?)
prevails over Cold.
Saltiness injures the Blood (bones?),
but sweetness prevails over saltiness.

THIS LAST SECTION ON COSMIC RESONANCES IN THE HUMAN body is likely to contain two scribal errors, both found in the last line: As I have marked in both cases by means of adding the corrected word with a question mark in parentheses, it is possible that *xuè* 血 (Blood) is a mistake for *gǔ* 骨 (bones), and that *zào* 燥 (Parching) is a mistake for *shī* 濕 (Dampness). The case for substituting bones for Blood is supported by the fact that the same passage in the *Tài Sù* has that character instead. If we are, however, to try and make sense of the text as it is written above, Gāo Shìzōng's commentary might help. For a longer discussion on the possible clinical significance and reasoning for the presence of Blood here as the physical constituent affected by Cold, see below.

* * *

Commentary By Gāo Shìzōng 高士宗

腎臟五臟之精，而屬於陰，故不言骨而言血。

土能勝水，當云濕勝寒，今云燥勝，以明寒濕同類，
燥土之氣，以勝水氣之寒也。

The Kidney stores the Essence of the Five Zàng Organs and is associated with Yīn. Therefore the text does not speak of the bones but speaks of the blood.

Earth is able to prevail over Water, and the text should say 'Dampness prevails over Cold' here. The reason why here it states instead that Parching prevails is that Cold and Dampness are clearly in the same category and that here we have the Qì of Parched Earth that can thereby prevail over the Cold of Water Qì.

* * *

Concluding Discussion of Sections 7–11

It is important to read the five sections above in the context of this chapter as a whole and in particular in response to the introductory first part of the Great Discourse. As such, these five passages constitute Qí Bó's answer to the Yellow Emperor's question about how "the sages of high antiquity discussed and patterned the human body in accordance with deeper organizing principles, arrayed and differentiated the *Zàng* and *Fǔ* Organs, and laid out the channels and vessels in a grid of vertical stems and horizontal branches." In response, Qí Bó here elucidates the fundamental resonances between the microcosm of the human body and the macrocosm of the natural environment in both Heaven and on Earth by listing specific connections between them. Still memorized by every serious student of Chinese medicine today, the five sections above introduce the following correlations for each of the Five Dynamic Agents (*wǔ xíng* 五行):

The cardinal directions (*fāng* 方):
east, south, center, west, and north,

The climatic factors (*qì* 氣):
Wind, Cold, Dampness, Dryness, and Cold,

The dynamic agents (*xíng* 行):
Wood, Fire, Earth, Metal, and Water,

The Flavors (*wèi* 味):
sour, bitter, sweet, acrid, and salty,

The *Zàng* Organs (*zàng* 臟):
Liver, Heart, Spleen, Lung, and Kidney,

The physical constituents (*tǐ* 體):
sinews, Blood/vessels, flesh, skin and body hair,
and bones and marrow,

THE MOTHER-CHILD RELATIONS IN THE CYCLE OF CREATION (*SHĒNG* 生):
Heart, Spleen, Lung, Kidney, Liver,

THE OPENINGS (*QIÀO* 竅):
eyes, tongue, mouth, nose, and ears

THE HUES (*SÈ* 色):
pale green, red, yellow, white, and black,

THE MUSICAL NOTES (*YĪN* 音):
jué, zhǐ, gōng, shāng, and yǔ,

THE SOUNDS OF THE HUMAN VOICE (*SHĒNG* 聲):
shouting, laughter, singing, coughing, and moaning,

THE PATHOLOGICAL MOVEMENTS (*BIÀN DÒNG* 變動):
clenching, mourning, dry heaving, coughing, and trembling,

THE WILLS, OFTEN REFERRED TO AS THE "FIVE EMOTIONS" (*ZHÌ* 志):
anger, happiness, ruminating, worry, and fear.

IN GENERAL, IT IS INTERESTING TO NOTE THE VARIOUS INTERACTIONS between the Five Dynamic Agents as outlined here. In the second to last association in each of the first lines of the five sections, the text mentions how the physical constituent associated with each Agent engenders the next Agent in accordance with the cycle of creation (*shēng* 生), such as the Liver's sinews engendering the Heart, the Heart's Blood engendering the Spleen, the Spleen's flesh engendering the Lung, etc. in what are clearly descriptions of physiological processes.

By contrast, the last sentence of each section discusses pathology, starting with the pathogenic effects of the emotions, since they stir the Qì and thereby endanger the normal harmonious relationships among the five agents. To counterbalance this imbalance, however, the text now brings in the cycle of restraint (*kè* 剋), stating that "grief prevails over anger," just like Lung-Metal is able to prevail over Liver-Wood in a physiological cycle of restraint. Similarly, the Lung's climate of Parching is able to mitigate the negative effects of pathological Liver-Wind, and its acrid Flavor is able to overcome the effects of excessive sourness. These five sections thereby indicate not only physiological relationships and normal correlations between the Five Agents in the microcosm of the human body and the external macrocosm when it is in perfect harmony and balance. In addition, these passages also offer advice to an educated person on how to mitigate potential negative effects from an excess of any one influence by availing oneself of the cycle of restraint. In this way, we can reestablish the necessary equilibrium between all five of these forces in their ever-changing constellations of Yīn-Yáng dynamics to counteract any excessive exposure of one force, whether from diet, climate, activity, emotion, or any other internal or external factor.

Placed perhaps intentionally between the description of healthy relationships in the first sentence and the discussion of pathology and treatment in the third sentence, the middle sentence provides important information for an astute physician or any person with sagely insights in terms of diagnosis, from facial complexion to the sound of the voice, unintentional pathological movements, and emotional expressions. It is for good reasons that these five paragraphs are quoted in any reputable foundational textbook of Chinese medicine to this day!

One interesting twist in this seemingly straightforward list, however, is introduced in the third lines of Sections Eight and Eleven: The other lines discuss injury to the physical constituent associated with that agent as being caused by an excess of its associated climatic factor and Flavor (i.e., Wind and sourness injuring the sinews, Dampness and sweetness injuring the flesh, and Cold and acridity injuring the skin and body hair). By contrast, Section Eight (on Heart-Fire) discusses the effect of Heat and bitterness on the Qì, while Section Eleven (on Kidney-Water) discusses the effect of Cold and saltiness on the Blood. Ordinarily, one would expect Blood to be associated more closely with the Heart (as explained in the first line of Section Eight where "the Heart engenders Blood," and through its association with the vessels as the physical constituent), while the Qì is generally associated with the Lung. Similarly, the climatic factor and Flavor associated with the Kidney (Cold and saltiness) should affect the bone and marrow, rather than the Blood! What are we to make of these inconsistencies? We can either explain them away as textual errors or we can take them seriously as reflections of clinical experience or different perspectives that occasionally override blind applications of so-called correlative thinking on the basis of the Five Dynamic Agents, in which case we have to pay extra attention to this information.

On a superficial level, it certainly makes practical clinical sense that the text emphasizes the dangers of excessive Cold and saltiness on the Blood, rather than on the deeper-lying bones, in the case of Section Eleven. And when we view Blood as fluid and recall the Kidney's association with Water, the negative effect of Cold on the free flow of fluids is obvious, since cold congeals fluids and inhibits their flow. Similarly, the Heart is in the upper body and the abode of the *Shén*, in charge of the ineffable Yáng aspects of the body that are represented by Qì in its opposition with Blood. And as Section Three above states, "Strong Fire consumes Qì… Strong Fire scatters Qì." Similarly, Section Four above states, "Cold injures the Form; Heat injures Qì."

Thus we only need to recall earlier discussions on Heat and Cold in the Great Discourse, and on their association with Yáng and Yīn respectively, and then relate that to the association of Qì with Yáng and Blood with Yīn, and this list once again makes perfect logical sense. What this passage demonstrates to me is the superimposed application of the vertical Kidney-Heart, Water-Fire, Yīn-Yáng axis over the five-fold cycle of the Five Dynamic Agents, which is bound to cause inconsistencies when looked at from one perspective, in order to make sense of it from another perspective, in the same way that the combination of Four Seasons and Five Agents (let alone the Six Qì that were introduced in the doctrine of the "Five Movements and Six Qì" (*wǔ yùn liù qì* 五運六氣) in subsequent centuries in such later chapters as *Sù Wèn* Chapter 66, which I have therefore cited above) is bound to cause incongruencies. When we encounter such apparent contradictions between individual lines within this chapter, or between different chapters in the *Huáng Dì Nèi Jīng*, it is always important to remember the early history of the text. Scholars have long used such internal contradictions as evidence that this chapter on its own and the text as a whole is a collage of many layers of sayings and teachings that had been memorized and transmitted orally for centuries before being committed to writing. In addition, these inconsistencies point to efforts already in the early texts to reconcile the strictures of correlative thinking in Five Agent theory with their clinical experience. As such, they can be viewed as proof that the authors of the *Néi Jīng* were far from automatic in their application of theory, even in this chapter devoted explicitly to Yīn-Yáng resonances. Instead, they crafted a body of literature that truly reflects their efforts to express their knowledge of the guiding principle operating in Heaven, as they saw it reflected in the realm of the human body.

Part Three

Attuning Yīn & Yáng

Section Twelve

故曰：天地者，萬物之上下也；陰陽者，血氣之男女也；左右者，陰陽之道路也；水火者，陰陽之徵兆也；陰陽者，萬物之能始也。

Gù yuē: Tiān dì zhě,
wàn wù zhī shàng xià yě;
yīn yáng zhě, xuè qì zhī nán nǚ yě;
zuǒ yòu zhě, yīn yáng zhī dào lù yě;
shuǐ huǒ zhě, yīn yáng zhī zhēng zhào yě;
yīn yáng zhě, wàn wù zhī néng shǐ yě.

Therefore, it is said:
'Heaven and Earth! They are the
above and below of the Myriad Things.
Yīn and Yáng! They are the
male and female of Blood and Qì.
Left and right! They are the
path of Yīn and Yáng.
Water and Fire! They are the evidence
and portents of Yīn and Yáng.
Yīn and Yáng, they are the
potential and the fetal beginning
of the Myriad Things.'

THIS SECTION CONSTITUTES QÍ BÓ'S CONCLUDING STATEMENT, to wrap up the list of resonances between Heaven, Earth, and Humanity that he has offered in the previous five sections. Let us not forget that he has been presenting this information in response to the Yellow Emperor's question about whether the ancient sages' mapping and structuring of the human body in resonance with the cosmic order is trustworthy. Once again, we encounter two lines here that could be the topic of a whole book on their own. Especially the second line is one that is often quoted by Chinese doctors and has been memorized by hundreds of generations of Chinese medicine doctors. After Qí Bó in his answer has first elucidated the correspondences between the human body and its Earthly and Heavenly environment in great detail in terms of the Five Dynamic Agents, he now changes tack to return to the main topic of the *Great Discourse*, the resonances of Yīn and Yáng. As such, he reiterates here the primacy of Yīn and Yáng as the "Dào of Heaven and Earth" and the fundamental model for comprehending and correlating change in the human body and the macrocosm.

To properly understand the present line, it is necessary to consider the different possibilities for interpreting paired noun phrases in literary Chinese. For this purpose, let us look at some common examples. Most directly, we can read a pair of two characters as simply a combination of two nouns in a relationship of coordination, such as the compound *xuè qì* 血氣, meaning "Blood AND Qì." A bit more complicated is the compound *jīng qì* 精氣, which can be interpreted variously as "Essence AND Qì" or, in a relationship of subordination, as "essential Qì." In other words, we can read it as a combination of two juxtaposed nouns of equal weight, or we can read it as a combination of what we would in English consider an adjective (精 "essential") and a noun, where the first character modifies the second character (氣 Qì). Lastly, a combination of two equally weighted nouns can assume a meaning that is greater than the sum of its parts. As such, the compound *tiān dì* 天地 "Heaven and Earth" means more than just heaven above and earth below, but refers to the universe as a whole, encompassing an unfathomable number of microcosms.

In the line above, it might be helpful to keep all of these possibilities in mind as we contemplate the meaning of the various noun combinations. As elsewhere in this chapter and the *Nèi Jīng* in general, more complicated physiological or pathological correlations are often preceded by more straight-forward and immediately graspable relationships in the natural world, at least from my personal perspective as a farmer. As such, the first pair, Heaven and Earth, is directly correlated with above and below, in a relationship that is intuitive to anybody who can look up at the sky and down at the dirt beneath their feet. It should be noted, however, that the two characters *shàng* 上 and *xià* 下, which I have translated literally as "the above and below" can also be read in the verbal sense of "ascending and descending," which would make this whole line say "Heaven and Earth! They are the ascending and descending of the Myriad Things." In a more elegant and less literal interpretation than what I have given above, we can also translate this entire phrase as "Heaven and Earth are what is above and below the Myriad Things."

The second correlation of Yīn and Yáng with "the male and female of Blood and Qì" takes Qí Bó's answer to a whole new level by addressing the relationship of Qì and Blood in the microcosm of the gendered human body. When first reading this line as a contemporary practitioner of Chinese medicine, it is tempting to interpret it in light of the standard treatment rule that became widely accepted and quoted from the Sòng period on:

Quotation from Chén Zìmíng[1]

大率治病，先論其所主。男子調其氣，女子調其血。

As a general guideline on treating disease, first discuss the aspect that [the patient] is ruled by. In men, attune their Qì; in women, attune their Blood.

Expressing the direct application of this common saying to the present line, Zhāng Jièbīn states simply that "Yáng constitutes Qì constitutes male, Yīn constitutes Blood constitutes female" (*yáng wéi qì wéi nán, yīn wéi xuè wéi nǚ* 陽為氣為男，陰為血為女). Nevertheless, we must remember that this gender-specific association of men with Qì and women with Blood was not stated, at least explicitly, prior to the Sòng dynasty. In that case, how else are we to read this statement that "Yīn and Yáng! They are the male and female of Blood and Qì"? Should we perhaps read "male and female" in a more general sense as the totality of all humans, in the same way that *tiān dì* 天地 means not just "Heaven and Earth" but the totality of all existence, or that *dà xiǎo* 大小 means not just "large and small" but "size"? And does the phrase "Blood and Qì" perhaps refer more generally to everything that moves inside the human body? And what does this expression actually mean, the "male and female of Qì and Blood"? To reference the second half of this Section below, the association of Yīn with being inside and with *shǒu* 守 ("safekeeping") and of Yáng with being outside and with *shǐ* 使, with being dispatched, running errands, acting as "envoy," is explicitly stated there. Reading that line in light of the traditional male and female roles in early Chinese society certainly sheds light on the two terms *shǒu* 守 "safekeeper" and

[1] *Chén Zìmíng* 《陳自明》, *Fùrén Dàquán Liáng Fāng* 婦人大全良方 (Excellent Comprehensive Formulas for Women).

shǐ 使 "executor." My best guess is that the "male and female" as the Yīn and Yáng aspects or functions of Blood and Qì can indeed be understood in light of the gendered roles of men and women in early Chinese society. Here it was normative behavior, especially among the elite literate scholar-bureaucrats who produced the *Néi Jīng*, for the men to leave the home and be active in the outside world, or in other words serve the government outside the home, often in far-away places, while the women stayed in the ancestral home of the family to bear and raise children and take care of elders in the extended patrilineal family. Unfortunately, it exceeds the limitations of this discussion here to explore the traditional associations of "male" and "female" in early Chinese society, ritual, and philosophy in detail, but this topic has been covered by many other scholars elsewhere. We can also just consider "male" and "female" here in terms of the natural reproductive functions and physiological (and pathological) associations of male and female bodies.

Similarly, I encourage the reader to contemplate the potential meanings of the following pairings from a variety of angles instead of just reading over them quickly. "Left and right"—is this a reference to the flow of Yīn and Yáng Qì in the human body? Or to the movement of heavenly bodies, the rising and setting sun and moon in particular, from the perspective of the ruler facing south? The answer should always be yes and yes, and to innumerable other microcosms that we simply may not think of in the current moment. According to Zhāng Zhìcōng's commentary, left and right are the manifestation of the diurnal circulation of Yīn and Yáng inside the human body.

"Water and Fire"—does this refer here to the vertical polarity between the Kidney and the Heart in their physiological functions, to the pathological manifestations of excess Yīn and Yáng, to the two most basic life-giving forces in the universe that form the foundation for all creation "under Heaven" in their downward-streaming and upward-flaring activity respectively, or does it serve as a short-hand for the Five Dynamic Agents 五行? Sometimes, I feel that the longer I contemplate the deeper meanings of a passage like this, the more I learn and yet the less I understand. Other times, I can see clearly that it does increase my comprehension of the Qì-Blood dynamic to utilize the lens of a Yīn-Yáng duality, whether they are in a healthy state of equilibrium or in a pathological imbalance with an excess of one or the other, along the lines suggested in this short passage.

Concerning the complicated phrase "evidence and portents of Yīn and Yáng"(*yīn yáng zhī zhēng zhào* 陰陽之徵兆), Wáng Bīng defines *zhēng* 徵 as *xìn* 信 in the sense of proof, evidence, or sign, while *zhào* 兆 is equated with *xiān* 先 "ahead of time." In other words, Yīn and Yáng, in their manifestation in the body as Cold and Heat, are the visible evidence, the manifestation, of the state of Yīn and Yáng in the body, as well as the advance signs of more serious illnesses to come if they are not addressed and corrected in due time. Alternatively, Zhāng Jièbīn explains:

Commentary by Zhāng Jièbīn 張介賓

征，証也。兆，見也。陰陽不可見，水火即其証而可見也。

Zhèng means evidence, and zhào means visible. Given that Yīn and Yáng are invisible, Water and Fire are their evidence and are visible.

The meaning of *néng shǐ* 能始, translated as "potential and fetal beginning" above, may appear straight-forward at first when translated as "able to begin." Nevertheless, it quickly becomes much more complicated when we contemplate a possible relationship between this line and the following passage from the Classic of Changes: Commentary on the Appended Phrases Yì Jīng (Classic of Changes) 《易經.系辭上傳》：乾知大始，坤作成物。乾以易知，坤以简能。 "Qián (symbolizes Heaven, which) directs the great beginnings of things; Kūn (symbolizes Earth, which) gives to them their completion. It is by the ease with which it proceeds that Qián directs (as it does), and by its unhesitating response that Kūn exhibits such ability" (Translation by James Legge). Read in this context, *néng* 能 refers to the Yīn potential that brings things to completion, while *shǐ* 始 refers to the generative force of Yáng. Another possibility would be that *néng* 能 is the hidden potential before it is made manifest, like the seed lying stored underground in winter, while *shǐ* 始 is the actual beginning, the fetus taking shape in the womb (hence the "woman" radical 女 of the character), or the seed that is beginning to sprout and burst through its hull. Interestingly enough, the parallel passage from *Sù Wèn* Chapter 66 cited below here replaces this phrase *néng shǐ* 能使 with *zhōng shǐ* 終始 "beginning and end" and relates it to Wood and Metal, and their respective actions of "sprouting" or giving birth (in the spring) and bringing to completion or maturing (in the fall). Other ways we might translate this phrase here are "potentiality and inception" or "capabilities and generative forces."

* * *

Quotation from Sù Wèn[2]

然天地者，萬物之上下也，左右者，陰陽之道路也。水火者，陰陽之徵兆也，金木者，生成之終始也。氣有多少，形有盛衰，上下相召，而損益彰矣。

This being so, Heaven and Earth are the above and below of the myriad things; left and right are the pathways of Yīn and Yáng; Water and Fire are the evidence and portents of Yīn and Yáng; Metal and Wood are the end and beginning of creating and bringing to completion. Qì can be profuse or scarce, the Form can be exuberant or weakened, above and below beckon each other, and losses and gains become ever more apparent!

* * *

[2] *Sù Wèn* 《素問》 Chapter 66, *Tiān Yuán Jì Dà Lùn* 天元紀大論 (Great Discourse on the Record of Heaven's Origin).

故曰：陰在內，陽之守也；陽在外，陰之使也。

Gù yuē:
Yīn zài nèi, yáng zhī shǒu yě;
yáng zài wài, yīn zhī shǐ yě.

Therefore, it is said:
'Yīn, being on the inside,
is the safekeeper of Yáng.
Yáng, being on the outside,
is the executor for Yīn.'"

This is one of the most important lines in the entire *Great Discourse* and perhaps in the *Yellow Emperor's Inner Classic* as a whole. It is also the perfect example of why it is essential to combine a thorough sinological training in the foundational historical literature with a clear understanding of grammar, as well as an appreciation for the meaning of any particular line in the context of its source text. Unschuld and Tessenow's translation of this line reads, "The Yīn is inside, it is the guardian of the Yáng. The Yáng is outside, it is employed by the Yīn."[3] While this translation dovetails the parallelism of the Chinese text nicely and certainly works grammatically, the last phrase, and especially the term "employed," reads a bit odd when we consider the nature and functioning of Yīn and Yáng in the universe and in the microcosm of the social realm, especially in the context of male-female relationships in a Confucian patriarchal and patrilineal system, or in their role in the human body, for that matter. The character *shǐ* 使 as a verb can mean "to cause somebody to do something," but conceptualizing Yáng as doing the bidding and following the orders of Yīn is problematic. Perhaps a better way to read it here is in the sense of "to make something happen," to "cause something to happen." As such, Yáng is the active half in the Yīn-Yáng pair, the entity that performs tasks, in the sense of the executive branch of government.

Quite differently, Elisabeth Rochat de la Vallée translates this line as "Yin is on the inside but Yáng keeps it there; Yáng is on the outside but Yīn sends it there."[4] She then explains that the association of "guard and defense" with Yáng Qì is related to its location on the outside (presumably through its role as *wèi qì* 衛氣, defense Qì). This interpretation of *shǒu* 守 as "keeping" and association of the term with the defensive role of Yáng unfortunately does not fit into the grammatical structure of the sentence and also misreads the meaning of *shǒu* 守 and its association with Yīn here. Similarly, Yīn is not the one doing the "sending" in the second half of the phrase. It is essential that we read *shǒu* 守 here not as "defense" in the sense of a guard on the

[3] Unschuld and Tessenow, 111.

[4] Rochat de la Vallée, 112.

exterior that protects the interior from outside invasions. As Rochat de la Vallée recognizes, that role is clearly a function associated with Yáng in Chinese medicine under the concept of *wèi Qì*. By contrast and as suggested by the etymology of the character 守, namely a hand 寸 under a roof 宀, the action of Yīn here connotes "keeping [something or somebody] close-by," attending to or keeping watch over, or in my translation above "safekeeping," which may sound similar in English to Unschuld and Tessenow's translation of "guard" but implies a completely different function in the present context. Here, it is better to think of Yīn in the role of the ideal wife who stays "under the roof," i.e. in the home, taking care of the young and old in the family, ensuring the survival and continuation of the lineage, and providing an anchor or safe harbor for the husband to return to and recharge, so that he can continue going out and performing his executive *shǐ* 使 functions.

Shǐ 使, on the other hand, can indeed mean "to send" or "to cause somebody to do something," or in Unschuld and Tessenow's translation "to employ." Nevertheless, I would be careful to translate this term here in the hierarchical sense of "servant" or "errand-runner." I read it as simply meaning that quiet Yīn, being on the inside, is relying on active Yáng to get things done on the outside, just like active Yáng on the outside is relying on quiet Yīn to provide a calm haven inside. Explaining this important phrase by means of the social relationship between husband and wife, as the much later *Lèi Jīng* 類經 (1624) quoted below does, is certainly one helpful way of envisioning the interaction between Yīn and Yáng.

* * *

Commentary by Zhāng Jièbīn 張介賓

陰性靜，故為陽之守；陽性動，故為陰之使。守者守於中，使者運於外。以法象言，則地守於中，天運於外；以人倫言，則妻守於中，夫運於外；以氣血言，則營守於中，衛運於外。故朱子曰：陽以陰為基，陰以陽為偶。

It is the nature of Yīn to be still, hence it serves as the safekeeper of Yáng. It is the nature of Yáng to be active, hence it serves as the executor of Yīn. "Safekeeper" means safekeeping in the center, and "executor" means moving around on the outside. Explaining this in terms of cosmic manifestations, Earth acts as safekeeper on the inside while Heaven moves around on the outside. In terms of human relationships, the wife acts as safekeeper in the center while the husband moves around on the outside. In terms of Qì and Blood, yíng provisioning safekeeps in the center while wèi defense moves around on the outside. For this reason, Zhū Xī said: "Yáng serves as the foundation for Yīn. Yīn serves as the counterpart to Yáng."

* * *

Nevertheless, we have to be very careful not to read our understanding of social relations and gendered hierarchies from Late Imperial China, or much less contemporary Western society, into a text that was compiled 1500 years earlier. To avoid this mistake, we can learn from recent work by historians in other fields of Chinese culture, such as Margaret J. Pearson. Her translation *The Original I Ching: An Authentic Translation of the Book of Changes Based on Recent Discoveries*, for example, presents a gender-neutral translation of the *Yì Jīng* that avoids the common pitfall of most other works on this topic to equate Yīn and Yáng automatically with female and male, respectively, and to project gender hierarchies from late Imperial China onto our reading of this ancient Zhōu dynasty text. Perhaps a better way to envision this relationship between quiet Yīn in the center and active Yáng on the outside here is the way in which the Heart rules the body through non-action by being situated calmly in the center, radiating *shén míng*, while the other organs carry out the bodily functions necessary to sustain the person and respond to the external environment.

Quotation from Sù Wèn[5]

心者，君主之官也，神明出焉。 肺者，相傳之官，治節出焉。
肝者，將軍之官，謀慮出焉。 膽者，中正之官，決斷出焉。
膻中者，臣使之官，喜樂出焉。 脾胃者，倉廩之官，五味出焉。
大腸者，傳道之官，變化出焉。 小腸者，受盛之官，化物出焉。
腎者，作強之官，伎巧出焉。 三焦者，決瀆之官，水道出焉。
膀胱者，州都之官，津液藏焉，氣化則能出矣。

THE HEART:
It occupies the office of the Sovereign.
Spirit luminosity stems from it.

THE LUNG:
It occupies the office of the Grand Councilor.
Order and good measure stem from it.

THE LIVER:
It occupies the office of the General.
Strategic planning stems from it.

THE GALLBLADDER:
It occupies the office of Impartiality and Rectitude.
Resolve and decision-making stem from it.

THE CENTER OF THE CHEST (DÀNZHŌNG):
It occupies the office of the Servant and Messenger.
Happiness and joy stem from it.

[5] *Sù Wèn* 《素問》 Chapter 8, *Líng Lán Mì Diǎn* 靈蘭秘典論 (Discourse on the Divine Orchid's Secret Canons).

The Spleen and Stomach:
They occupy the office of the Granary.
The five flavors stem from it.

The Large Intestine:
It occupies the office of Conveyance.
Gradual and substantive change stem from it.

The Small Intestine:
It occupies the office of Receiving and Containment.
The transformation of [ingested] matter stems from it.

The Kidney:
It occupies the office of Forceful Action.
Ingenuity and acumen stem from it.

The Triple Burner:
It occupies the office of Dredging and Draining.
[Free flow in] the water ways stems from it.

The Bladder:
It occupies the office of Metropolis Surrounded by Water.
The fluids are stored inside it and are able to emerge as
the result of qì transformation.

Section Thirteen

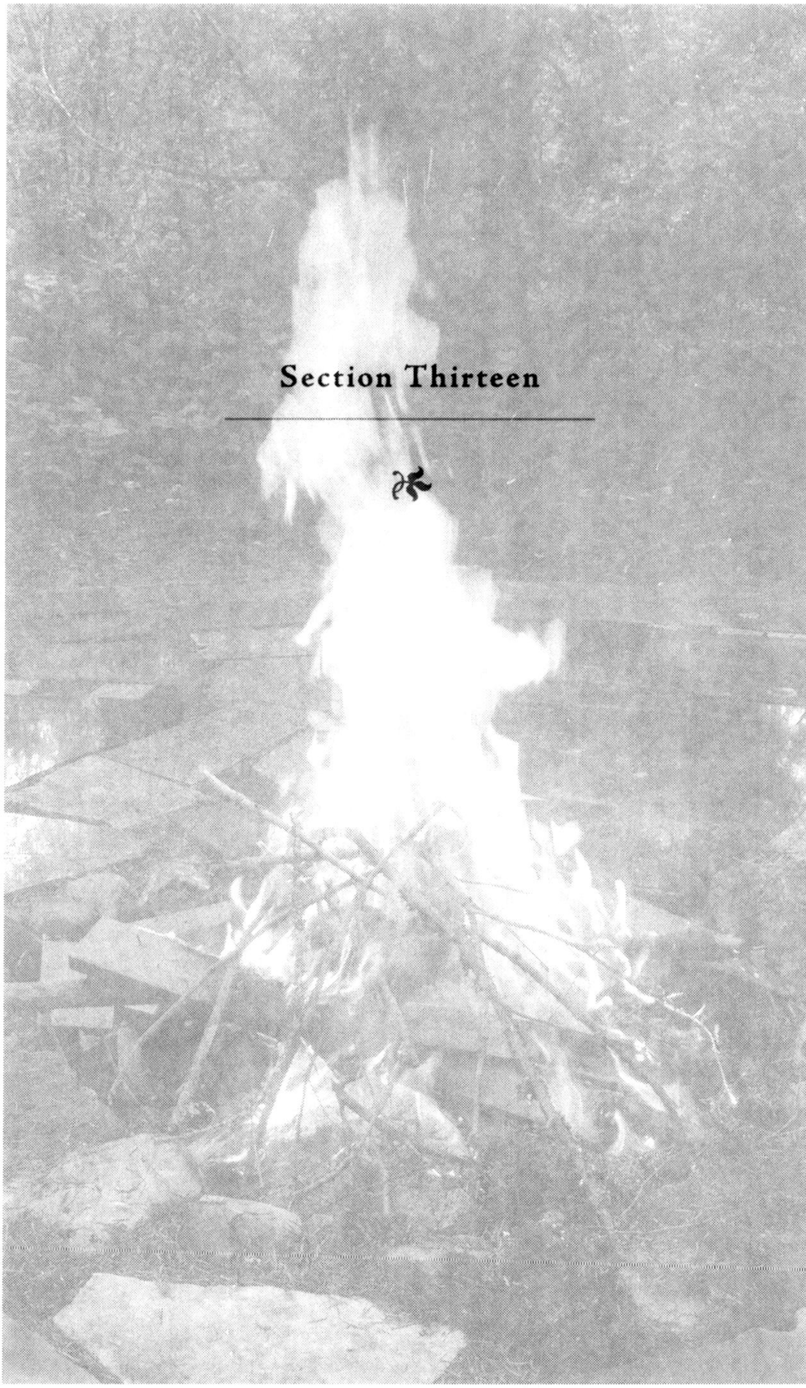

帝曰：法陰陽奈何？
岐伯曰：陽勝則身熱，腠理閉，喘粗為之俯仰，汗不出而熱，齒乾以煩冤腹滿死，能冬不能夏。

Dì yuē: Fǎ yīn yáng nài hé?

Qí Bó yuē: Yáng shèng zé shēn rè, còu lǐ bì, chuǎn cū wèi zhī fǔ yǎng, hàn bù chū ér rè, chǐ gān yǐ fán yuān fù mǎn sǐ, néng dōng bù néng xià.

The Emperor asked: "How do we go about conforming to Yīn and Yáng?"

Qí Bó said: "Prevalence of Yáng results in generalized Heat, closing of the texture lines of the skin and flesh, coarse panting and bending the body forward and backward as a result, sweat failing to exit followed by Heat, dryness of the teeth and therefore vexation and distress, fullness in the abdomen, and [then] death. [Such patients] can endure winter but not summer.

In the previous section, Qí Bó has emphatically affirmed that Yīn and Yáng are not only the key operating principle or Dào in the universe that "makes the world go 'round," but also the most fundamental paradigm for grasping the resonances between the macrocosm and the microcosm of the human body. Now the Yellow Emperor is asking for concrete details to apply this cosmic pattern to medical practice: What does a prevalence of Yīn or Yáng in the body look like in terms of clinical diagnosis? What are the pathological changes resulting from a disturbed equilibrium and an excess of one and deficiency of the other? Qí Bó is happy to provide the answer with this passage. In the commentary cited below, Gāo Shìzōng elaborates on the clinical reasoning behind the symptoms listed by Qí Bó:

* * *

Commentary by Gāo Shìzōng 高士宗

陽勝則火熱有餘，而身熱，熱氣在表，則腠理閉；熱氣在裡，則喘粗。表裡皆病，則為之俯仰，汗不出而內外皆熱也。齒干，津液竭也。以煩冤腹滿死者，津液既竭，又心煩而屈抑不舒，腹滿而土氣內絕，故死。雖不即死也，能冬不能夏。冬時寒冷，陽勝可容，夏時炎暑，不堪煎厥矣。

A prevalence of Yáng means that there is a surplus of Fire and Heat. As a result, we see generalized Heat. When the Heat Qì is in the exterior, the texture lines of the skin and flesh close up, and when the Heat Qì is in the interior, there is coarse panting. When both the exterior and interior suffer from illness, this results in bending backward and forward, failure to sweat, and Heat both on the inside and on the outside. Dryness of the teeth means that the fluids are exhausted. The reason why this leads to vexation and distress, abdominal fullness, and death is that the full exhaustion of the fluids causes Heart vexation and subsequent bending, restraint and discomfort, as well as abdominal fullness and subsequent internal expiry of Earth Qì, and therefore death. Even when this situation does not immediately cause death, it is tolerable in winter but intolerable in summer. In the freezing cold of winter a prevalence of Yáng can be accommodated, but in the scorching heat of summer [the patient] cannot bear Frying Reversal.

陰勝則身寒汗出，身常清，數栗而寒，寒則厥，厥則腹滿死，能夏不能冬。

此陰陽更勝之變，病之形能也。

Yīn shèng zé shēn hán hàn chū,
shēn cháng qīng, shuò lì ér hán,
hán zé jué, jué zé fù mǎn sǐ,
néng xià bù néng dōng.

Cǐ yīn yáng gèng shèng zhī
biàn, bìng zhī xíng néng yě.

Prevalence of Yīn results in generalized Cold, sweating, constant coolness of the body and frequent shivering followed by cold, cold then resulting in Reversal, Reversal then resulting in fullness in the abdomen, and [then] death. [Such patients] are able to endure summer but not winter.

These are the alterations [that result from] Yīn and Yáng prevailing over each other, and the Forms and potential [complications] of their pathologies."

Three of the symptoms mentioned in this passage require additional explanation: Both characters in the expression *fán yuān* 煩冤 ("vexation and distress") refer to feelings of mental agony that can perhaps be explained by the etymology of the characters: *Fán* 煩 is a combination of "fire" and "head," the meaning of which is self-explanatory. *Yuān* 冤 depicts a rabbit under a roof. Hence we can deduce that the character may here refer to an experience of illness that recalls the tormented panicking and distress of a caged rabbit. Most commentators read the phrase here simply as "vexation and oppression" (*fán mèn* 煩悶). Zhāng Jièbīn equates *yuán* 冤 with *yù ér luàn* 鬱而亂, the mental confusion resulting from the gloomy oppression felt in an overgrown entangled thicket with no way out (often mistakenly translated as "depression").

For the etymology and meaning of *jué* 厥 ("Reversal"), see my note above in Section Five, on page 134. In that context, some commentators equate the term with *nì* 逆 (countercurrent). Considering the clinical application of the line in the present context of Yīn prevalence causing cold, this equation is inadequate here. As stated in the previous discussion of *jué* 厥, these two characters do have overlapping meanings but are by no means identical. Here it is clear that the term includes the clinical symptom of cold in the extremities, referred to in Chinese as *sì zhī jué lěng* 四肢厥冷 (reversal cold in the four limbs).

The last symptom that requires additional explanation here is "constant coolness of the body" (*shén cháng qīng* 身常清). Readers who are not interested in philological ruminations may want to skip the following paragraphs and continue reading with the translation of Section Fourteen. In medical literature, the character *qīng* 清 can have three different meanings, all of which are found in various passages in the *Nèi Jīng*. How we decide to understand it in a specific passage depends on the grammar of the sentence, placement of the character in the text, content of the line, and context of the passage. As the first step in approaching a questionable character in a text, we look for possible character combinations, juxtapositions, parallel constructions, or intentional contrasts with other characters with a clearer meaning, to point us towards one particular meaning among the various possibilities. When we find such a pairing, the meaning tends to be immediately clear, which we can usually see supported by the fact that all commentators and mainstream translators read it in the same way.

In passages where this approach proves impossible because the character stands on its own, we must contemplate the content of the statement, whether cosmological, philosophical, or clinical, and the author's possible intentions with the phrase, line, and whole paragraph that the character occurs in. Here it is essential that we have familiarized ourselves with the particular terminology used in the text and with the author's style and cultural background. Thus a definition that we find in a Chinese-English dictionary may or may not be an appropriate option in a particular text, or it may have a different connotation in English that can lead us astray. A good example of this kind of danger is the choice of the English "guard" as a translation for *shǒu* 守 ("safe keeping") in the previous section that discusses Yīn being the safekeeper of Yáng instead of its external defense force. Here we must remember the inherent limitations of English-language dictionaries of literary Chinese, which can only take us so far. There is a reason why Chinese and Japanese dictionaries like the *Hànyǔ Dà Cídiǎn* 漢語大辭典 and the *Dai Kanwa Jiten* 大漢和辭典 consist of dozens of volumes with literally tens of thousands of pages, where each definition of a character is accompanied by historical citations that include the earliest and most relevant occurrences in the received literature. As any traditional sinologist, whether Chinese, Japanese, Korean, or from any other country, knows, the ability to read classical Chinese texts of any genre is developed slowly over decades of reading the literature in one's field of specialization, in addition to the standard classics that the authors of this literature would have been familiar with.

One last tool in our translator's toolbox is often the hardest one to use because it is the least rational: By studying the etymology and "sphere of meaning" of any character, its essence, if you will, that forms the core or root from which all possible English meanings are derived, we are often able to intuit what the meaning of a character in a particular context may be, even if none of the English dictionary definitions fit easily. So it is possible, for a character like Dào 道 or *lǐ* 理, that we develop an intuitive sense of the meaning of the character and can grasp what the author of a particular passage is wanting to express, even if we are unable to put our own understanding into English, simply because the English language does not have the vocabulary to express it adequately. Beginning students of classical Chinese often turn straight to the tool of etymology and ignore the first and second steps above. On the one hand, it is commendable to analyze a character's etymology instead of just picking a random definition from the list of possible meanings in English dictionaries. On the other hand, though, etymology is a complicated and specialized field of study, and the handy explanations of characters provided in especially English-language printed or on-line dictionaries are often wrong or overly simplifying. Moreover, we need to remember that etymology is only one tool among many that can shed light on a character's meaning in any one context and may or may not be relevant for the character's usage many centuries later.

Let us see how these approaches might contribute to our understanding of *qīng* 清 in the passage above from the *Great Treatise*: *Yīn sheng zé shén hán hàn chū, shén cháng qīng, shuò lì ér hán* 《陰勝則身寒汗出，身常清，數栗而寒。》 Yīn prevailing results in generalized cold, sweating, constant coolness of the body and frequent shivering followed by cold. In the *Nèi Jīng*, the character *qīng* 清 is used in three different ways.

First, it can mean "clear" or "pure," in reference to the top layer of a fluid or other substance in which impurities have settled to the bottom. Here it is often contrasted with *zhuó* 濁 "turbid," "murky," or "muddy." Examples for this usage are found in two passages from this chapter, the first from the introduction, the second from Section Seventeen below:

Quotations from Sù Wèn[1]

寒極生熱，熱極生寒。寒氣生濁，熱氣生清。清氣在下，
則生飧泄；濁氣在上，則生䐜脹。...故清陽為天，濁陰為地。

Extremes of Cold engender Heat; extremes of Heat engender Cold. Cold Qì engenders turbidity; Heat Qì engenders clearness. When clear Qì is located below, it engenders diarrhea with undigested food particles; when turbid Qì is located above, it engenders swelling and distention... Therefore, clear Yáng constitutes Heaven; turbid Yīn constitutes Earth."

清陽上天，濁陰歸地... 善診者，察色按脈，先別陰陽；審清濁，而知部分。

Clear Yáng rises to Heaven, turbid Yīn homes to the Earth... Practitioners who are skilled at diagnosis investigate the complexion and palpate the pulse, to first differentiate Yīn and Yáng. By examining the clear and the turbid, they know the specific location and level [of the disease]...

A SECOND MEANING OF *QĪNG* 清 , ALSO AS "CLEAR" OR "PURE," SOUNDS identical to the first meaning, just like in Chinese, but here refers to a state of mind that is free from impurities and distractions. This meaning is most apparent in passages that contain the compound *qīngjìng* 清靜 "clear and still," and is most prevalent in the more philosophical chapters at the beginning of the *Nèi Jīng*.

[1] *Sù Wèn* 《素問》 Chapter 5, See Sections 1 and 2 above.

⁂

Quotation from Sù Wèn[2]

秋三月，此謂容平，天氣以急，地氣以明，早臥早起，與雞俱興，
使志安寧，以緩秋刑，收斂神氣，使秋氣平，無外其志，使肺氣清，
此秋氣之應，養收之道也。 。。。 天氣清
淨，光明者也，藏德不止，故不下也。

The three months of autumn: This is the season referred to as 'receiving and balance.' The Qì of Heaven thereby is harsh, and the Qì of Earth thereby is bright. Go to bed early and rise early, stirring with the chickens! Let your will be at ease and tranquil, in order to relax the punishments of autumn! Gather in and restrain your spirit and your Qì, to make the Qì of autumn balanced. Do not allow your will to stray outside and thereby make your Lung Qì clear. This is responding to the Qì of autumn and the way of nurturing gathering in. ...This is because the Qì of heaven is marked by a state of clarity and stillness, and by radiant brightness. It ceaselessly keeps its power stored/hidden and therefore does not descend.

Quotation from Sù Wèn[3]

蒼天之氣，清淨則志意治，順之則陽氣固，
雖有賊邪，弗能害也。此因時之序。

Concerning the Qì of the far distant sky, when it is clear and still, the will and intention are in good order. When you are in alignment with it, the Yáng Qì is secure, and even though there may be robbers and evils present, they will be unable to cause harm. This is due to being in accord with the progression of the seasons."

[2] *Sù Wèn* 《素問》 Chapter 2, *Sì Qì Tiáo Shén Lùn* 四氣調神論 (Discourse on Attuning the *Shén* with the Four Qì).

[3] *Sù Wèn* 《素問》 Chapter 3, *Shēng Qì Tōng Tiān Lùn* 生氣通天論 (Discourse on the Vital Qì Connecting With Heaven).

The third possibility for interpreting *QĪNG* 清 is one that is not listed in even the best English dictionary for classical Chinese, Paul W. Kroll's *Student's Dictionary of Classical and Medieval Chinese*, but found in large Chinese-Chinese dictionaries and attested in historical literature. In the medical context, this meaning is also universally accepted by historical and contemporary commentators and translators in numerous *Nèi Jīng* passages alone. According to the vast majority of Chinese commentators, this is the correct meaning of *qīng* 清 in the present context. I follow their lead for the simple reason that it makes immediate sense. In addition to the meanings of "pure" and "clear" above, the character 清 can be used interchangeably with its close relative 凊, which means "cool" and is almost identical except that the "water" radical (three dots on the side of the character) is replaced with the "ice" radical (two dots). Here are just two unequivocal examples of this usage from the *Nèi Jīng*.

* * *

Quotation from Sù Wèn[4]

青脈之至也，長而左右彈，有積氣在心下。。。名曰肝痺。
得之寒濕，與疝同法。腰痛足清頭痛。

If a green-blue [complexion is accompanied by] a pulse's arrival that is extended and pellet-like on the left and right, there is accumulated Qì below the Heart...which is called "Liver bì impediment." It is contracted from Cold-Dampness and the model is identical with shàn mounding. [You will see] lumbar pain, cool feet, and headache.

* * *

[4] *Sù Wèn* 《素問》 Chapter 10, *Wǔ Zàng Shēng Chéng* 五臟生成 (The Formation of the Five Zàng Organs).

Quotation from Sù Wèn[5]

諸過者切之，澀者陽氣有餘也，滑者陰氣有餘也。陽氣有餘為身熱無汗，陰氣有餘為多汗身寒， 。。。。推而外之，內而不外，有心腹積也。推而內之，外而不內，身有熱也。推而上之，上而不下，腰足清也。

In all cases of excess, take the pulse. If it is rough, Yáng Qì has excess; if it is slippery, Yīn Qì has excess. Excess of Yáng Qì means generalized heat without sweating; excess of Yīn Qì means profuse sweating and generalized cold... If you push the vessel to the outside and it stays inside and does not move outside, this means accumulation in the Heart and abdomen. If you push it upward and it moves upward and does not descend, this means ***coolness in the lumbus and feet****.*

Two other short passages that clearly use the character *qīng* 清 in the sense of "cool" are as follows: 《心瘧者，令人 煩心甚，欲得清水，反寒多，不甚熱，刺手少陰。》 "As for Heart malaria, [this condition] causes patients to suffer from vexation in the Heart that is severe. They want to obtain cool water, but contrary [to expectations] present with increased cold and not great Heat. Needle the hand Shàoyīn... (*Sù Wèn* Chapter 36), and 《刺諸熱者，如以手探湯；刺寒清者，如人不欲行。》 "Needling the various Heat conditions is like testing boiling water with one's hand. Needling cool and cold conditions is like a person who does not want to leave...." (*Líng Shū* 靈樞 Chapter 1). The above-quoted passage in *Sù Wèn* Chapter 17 in particular repeats the association of excess Yīn Qì with generalized cold and sweating, and then coolness as an effect of the discharge of sweat, which we also see mentioned in the line in question above. The

[5] *Sù Wèn* 《素問》 Chapter 17, *Mài Yào Jīng Wēi Lùn* 脈要精微論 (Discourse on the Crucial Subtleties of the Pulse).

other examples here merely show that *qīng* 清 is indeed commonly used with the meaning of "cool" by the authors of the *Nèi Jīng.*

To return to our discussion of *Sù Wèn* 5, I read 能 *néng* in the compound *xíng néng* 形能, which I have translated as "Forms and potential [complications]" in the previous passage above, literally here as the "potential" of the disease. Many other commentators, however, interpret it here as a different character: *tài* 態, meaning "appearance" or "condition." Given the date of the compilation of the *Sù Wèn*, a time when it was very common to leave out or exchange radicals, either reading of this line is possible.

Section Fourteen

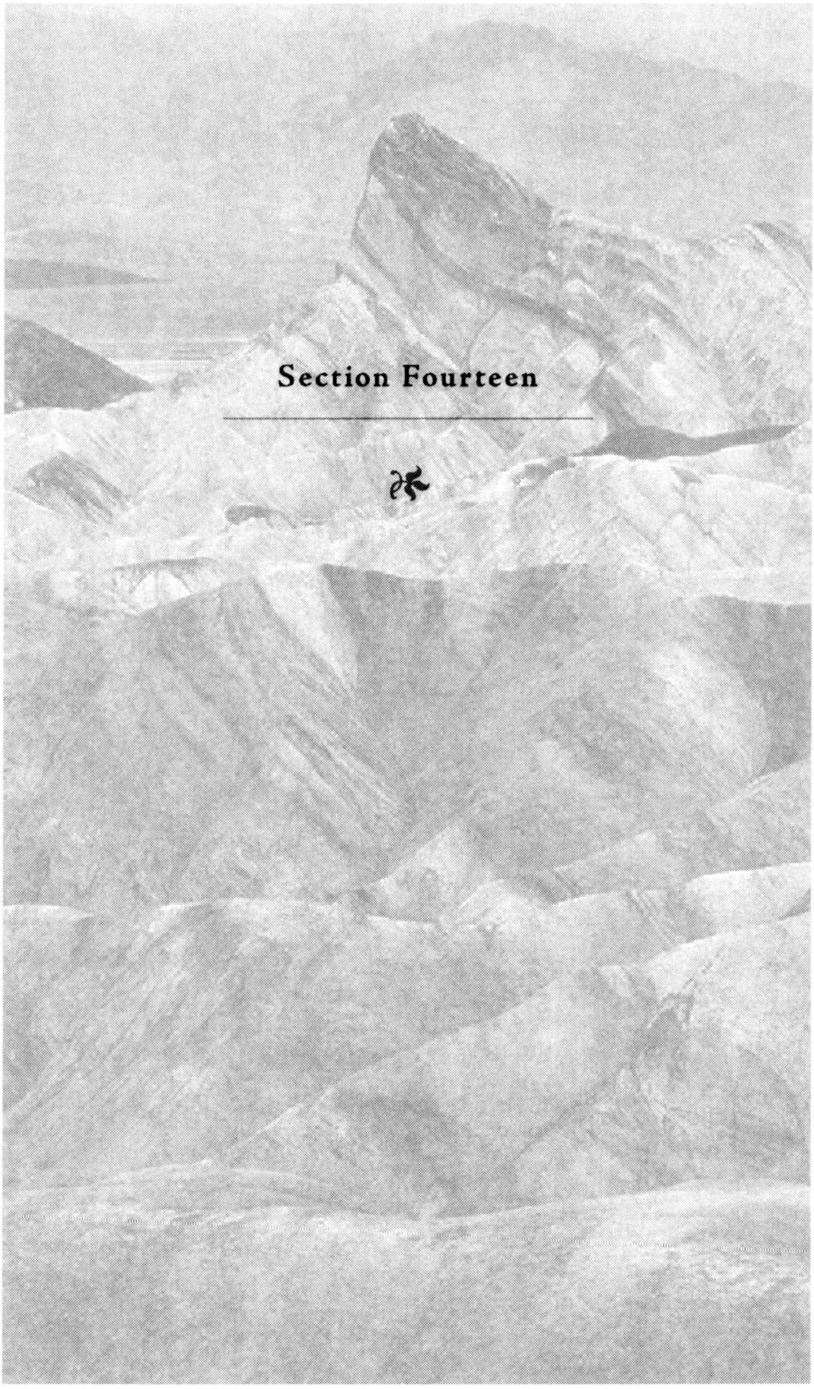

帝曰：調此二者奈何？

岐伯曰：能知七損八益，則二者可調；不知用此，則早衰之節也。

Dì yuē: Tiáo cǐ èr zhě nài hé?

Qí Bó yuē: Néng zhī qī sǔn bā yì, zé èr zhě kě tiáo; bù zhī yòng cǐ, zé zǎo shuāi zhī jié yě.

The Emperor asked: "How do we go about attuning these two?"

Qí Bó said: "If you are able to know the Seven Detriments and Eight Benefits, then these two can be attuned. If you do not know how to employ these, it will result in the limitations of premature decrepitude.

Whenever *Jīng* Essence is scarce, illness results. When it is all used up, death results. Restraint and caution are an absolute necessity. To frequently have intercourse and occasionally have a single leak causes Essence Qì to grow alongside this practice, and this cannot make such a person empty and harm them. But to frequently have intercourse followed by a discharge of Essence so that the Essence is unable to grow and increase results in moving Essence being all used up![1]

After Qí Bó has explained to the Yellow Emperor what an excess of Yīn and an excess of Yáng look like in the human body in the previous section, the Yellow Emperor is now ready to turn from diagnosis to treatment. Given the context, it is clear that "these two" (*cǐ èr* 此二) here refers to Yīn and Yáng, the topic of the preceding paragraph.

Commentators have long argued over the meaning of *qī sǔn bā yì* 七損八益, which most literally translates as "seven decreases and eight increases," but is here rendered as "Seven Detriments and Eight Benefits" for reasons that will become apparent shortly. *Sǔn* 損 means "to subtract," but also carries the meaning of "injury" in medical literature, while *yì* 益 means "to add," but in medical contexts also "to boost" or "to benefit," as in the common phrase *yì qì* 益氣, "to boost Qì." Historically, most commentators have read the expression here as referring to the description of female and male developmental processes in *Sù Wèn* Chapter 1 (Discourse on Heavenly Perfection in the Ancient Past 《上古天真論》) in multiples of seven and eight, respectively. While the number seven in girls is associated with a decrease, namely the loss of menstrual fluids, they argue, the number eight in boys is associated with an increase, namely the exuberance of Essence Qì.

[1] Táo Hóngjǐng 陶弘景, *Yǎng Xìng Yán Mìng Lù* 《養性延命錄》 (Record on Nurturing the Inner Nature and Extending Destiny), 6th century CE.

Quotation from Sù Wèn[2]

岐伯曰：女子七歲腎氣盛，齒更髮長；二七而天癸至，任脈通，太衝脈盛，月事以時下，故有子；三七腎氣平均，故真牙生而極；四七筋骨堅，髮長極，身體盛壯；五七陽明脈衰，面始焦，髮始墮；六七三陽脈衰於上，面皆焦，髮始白；七七任脈虛，太衝脈衰少，天癸竭，地道不通，故形壞而無子也。

丈夫八歲腎氣實，髮長齒更；二八腎氣盛，天癸至，精氣溢寫，陰陽和，故能有子；三八腎氣平均，筋骨勁強，故真牙生而長極；四八筋骨隆盛，肌肉滿壯；五八腎氣衰，發墮齒槁；六八陽氣衰竭於上，面焦，髮鬢頒白；七八肝氣衰，筋不能動，天癸竭，精少，腎藏衰，形體皆極；八八則齒發去。

Qí Bó said: "When girls are in their seventh year of life, their Kidney Qì begins to flourish, their teeth change, and the hair on their head grows long. In their fourteenth year, the tiānguǐ arrives, the flow in the Rènmài penetrates, the great Chōngmài is exuberant, and the menses descend in a timely manner. Therefore they can have children. In their twenty-first year, the Kidney Qì is balanced and even. Therefore the true [i.e., wisdom] teeth are born and growth reaches its limit. In their twenty-eighth year, the sinews and bones are firm, the growth of head hair has reached its limit, and the body is exuberant and strong. In their thirty-fifth year, the Yángmíng vessel weakens, the face becomes scorched, and the hair begins to fall out. In their forty-second year, the three Yáng vessels weaken above, the face is scorched all over, and the head hear begins to turn white. In their forty-ninth year, the Rènmài is empty, the great Chōngmài is weakened and reduced, the tiānguǐ is exhausted, and the pathways of the earth are impenetrable. Therefore their Form disintegrates, and they can no longer have children.

Regarding men, in the eighth year of life, the Kidney Qì is replete, the hair on the head grows long, and the teeth change. In their sixteenth year, the Kidney Qì is exuberant, the tiānguǐ arrives, Essence Qì spills over and drains out, and Yīn and

[2] *Sù Wèn* 《素問》 Chapter 1, *Shàng Gǔ Tiān Zhēn Lùn* 上古天真論 (Discourse on the Heavenly Truth in Ancient Antiquity).

Yáng harmonize [i.e., sexual intercourse takes place]. Therefore they are able to have children. In their twenty-fourth year, the Kidney Qì is balanced and even, and the sinews and bones are robust and strong. Therefore the true teeth emerge and growth reaches its limit. In their thirty-second year, the sinews and bones are abundant and exuberant and the flesh is full and strong. In their fortieth year, the Kidney Qì weakens, the head hair falls out, and the teeth wither. In their forty-eighth year, the Yáng Qì is weakened and exhausted above, the face becomes scorched, and the hair on the head and temples turns grey and white. In their fifty-sixth year, the Liver Qì weakens, the sinews are no longer able to move [freely], the tiānguǐ is exhausted, Essence is reduced, the Kidney is weakened, and the body is all used up. In their sixty-fourth year, they lose their teeth and head hair.

THE INTERPRETATION OF "SEVEN DETRIMENTS AND EIGHT BENEFITS" in terms of the aging cycles of women and men (or more literally "decreases" and "increases") is exemplified by Wáng Bīng's commentary:

Commentary by Wáng Bīng 王冰

調謂順天癸性，而治身之血氣精氣也。用謂房色。女子以七七為天癸之終，丈夫以八八為天癸之極，然知八可益，知七可損，則各隨氣分修養天真，終其天年以度百歲。內耗故陰減，中乾故氣力始衰。

"Attune" refers to the nature of the tiānguǐ and the proper management of the body's Blood Qì and Essence Qì. "Employ" refers to sexual intercourse. Women experience the end of their tiānguǐ at seven times seven (i.e. 49), and men experience the limit of their tiānguǐ at eight times eight (i.e. 64). This being so, if you know that the eight can be increased, and know that the seven can be decreased, then you can cultivate and nurture Heavenly perfection, each person according to their Qì, and live out your Heavenly life span to measure a hundred years of age. Internal consumption causes a reduction of Yīn; dryness in the center causes the debilitation of the life force to begin.

Nevertheless, this gendered association of men with increase and women with decrease has never made a whole lot of sense to me since men lose their Essence (*jīng* 精) in adulthood just like women lose their Blood, while during sexual intercourse women actually gain their male partner's Essence in perhaps a slightly more substantial way than men gain a female partner's. Additionally, *Sù Wèn* Chapter 1 also describes women's sexual maturity as an abundance in the Chōngmài ("The rènmài flows freely and the great Chōngmài is abundant" 任脈通，太衝脈盛). Other commentators have suggested that we read the phrase here as simply referring to the need to understand the various states of excess and insufficiency or the therapeutic practices that take away (in the case of excess) and supplement (in the case of deficiencies). Zhāng Jièbīn's commentary is a good illustration of the way in which this line has come to be commonly interpreted in late imperial China.

* * *

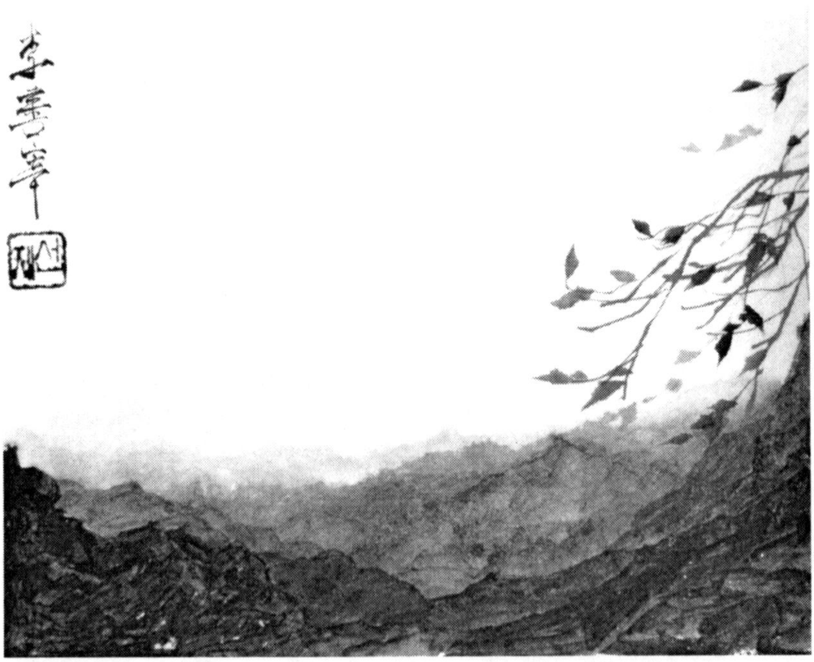

* * *

Commentary by Zhāng Jièbīn 張介賓

上文言陰陽之變病，此言死生之本原也。七為少陽之數，八為少陰之數。七損者言陽消之漸，八益者言陰長之由也。夫陰陽者，生殺之本始也，生從乎陽，陽不宜消也；死從乎陰，陰不宜長也。使能知七損八益之道，而得其消長之幾，則陰陽之柄，把握在我，故二者可調，否則未央而衰矣。

愚按：陰陽二氣，形莫大乎天地，明莫著乎日月。雖天地為對待之體，而地在天中，順天之化；日月為對待之象，而月得日光，賴日以明。此陰陽之征兆，陰必以陽為主也。故陽長則陰消，陽退則陰進，陽來則物生，陽去則物死，所以陰邪之進退，皆由乎陽氣之盛衰耳。故生氣通天等論皆專重陽氣，其義可知。

When the text above speaks of the pathological changes of Yīn and Yáng, this refers to the source of life and death. Seven is the number of Shàoyáng and eight is the number of Shàoyīn. The Seven Decreases refers to the gradual vanishing of Yáng, while the Eight Increases refers to the cause of Yīn growing. Now the reason why Yīn and Yáng are the root and beginning of life and death is that birth proceeds from Yáng and Yáng therefore should not vanish, while death proceeds from Yīn and Yīn therefore should not grow. If we are able to know the Dào of the Seven Decreases and Eight Increases and obtain the portents of their vanishing and growth, then the handle [to manage] Yīn and Yáng lies firmly in our own hands, and these two can therefore be attuned. Otherwise decrepitude awaits before the end.

I comment: In terms of the two Qì of Yīn and Yáng, no Form is greater than Heaven and Earth, and no brightness is more apparent than the sun and the moon. Even though heaven and Earth are two bodies opposite each other, Earth is in the middle of Heaven and follows along with the changes of Heaven. The sun and the moon are two manifestations opposite each other, and yet the moon receives the rays of the sun and depends on the sun for its brightness. These are the signs and portents of Yīn and Yáng, and Yīn must take Yáng as its ruler. For this reason, when Yáng grows, Yīn vanishes, and when Yáng retreats, Yīn advances. When Yáng arrives, things are born, and when Yáng leaves, things die. For this reason the advance and retreat of Yīn evil is all caused by the exuberance or debilitation of Yáng Qì. For this reason, Discourses like "Vital Qì Connecting with Heaven" (Sù Wèn Chapter 3) emphasize Yáng Qì specifically, and their meaning can be understood from this.

* * *

Note that the valuation of Yáng over Yīn that is expressed so strongly in this commentary on the passage above was a commonly accepted perspective in late imperial China, both in medicine and in the culture at large, but is not found anywhere in the original passage. As already stated above, we have to carefully avoid reading later theories and perspectives into early Chinese medical literature that might actually be talking about something completely unrelated. But then how are we to understand this expression "Seven Decreases and Eight Increases" and where are we to turn for a solution? The discovery of a text titled *Tiān Xià Zhì Dào Tán* 《天下至道談》(Discussion of the Ultimate Dào Under Heaven) among the Mǎwángduī 馬王堆 medical manuscripts, which predate 168 BCE, has forced us to revise all these guesses and read the phrase as a clear reference to the intentional cultivation of Qì during sexual intercourse. That text clearly spells out the meaning of each of the Eight Benefits and Seven Detriments beyond doubt:

* * *

Quotation from Tiān Xià Zhì Dào Tán[3]

八益：一日治氣，二日致沫，三日知時，四日畜氣，五日和沫，六日竊積氣，七日待贏，八日定傾。七損：一日閉，二日泄，三日竭，四日勿，五日煩，六日絕，七日費。

The Eight Benefits: To manage Qì, to make fluid arrive, to know timing, to amass Qì, to harmonize the fluids, to steal Qì, to await gain, and to secure against getting

[3] *Tiān Xià Zhì Dào Tán* 《天下至道談》(Discussion of the Ultimate Dào Under Heaven).

overturned. The Seven Detriments: Closure, leakage, exhaustion, inability, vexation, being cut off, and overconsumption.

* * *

In language that is strikingly similar to the passage above, the text issues this stern warning before presenting this list: "If you are unable to employ these, at the age of forty, Yīn Qì will be halved; at the age of fifty, your daily activities will have weakened; at the age of sixty, your ears and eyes lose their acuity; at the age of seventy, the lower body withers and the upper body is shed, the sexual organs become useless, and fluids and tears pour out.[4]"

It is widely attested, not only from the Mǎwángduī medical manuscripts but also from received literature even as late Sūn Sīmiǎo's 孫思邈 Qiān Jīn Fāng 千金方 from the seventh century, that sexual intercourse was one of the most important practices with which at least the literate elite, if not the general population, actively and intentionally cultivated longevity in the "Dào of nurturing life" (*yǎng shēng zhī dào* 養生之道). Referred to euphemistically and tellingly as "harmonizing Yīn and Yáng" *hé yīn yáng* 和陰陽 (or "matching Yīn and Yáng" 合陰陽), whole texts were written, in this early period exclusively from the male authors' perspective, about the potential benefits but also dangers of this activity in a man's life, which therefore had to be executed with utmost care and precision. Thus it makes perfect sense here that Qí Bó answers the Yellow Emperor's question on how to attune Yīn and Yáng with a reference to the specific risks and benefits that could result from the improper or proper performance of such a powerful activity. Since this text is written by and for men, it also makes sense here that ignorance of this practice will result in premature aging at the tender age of five times eight.

The inability to understand and employ these "Seven Detriments and Eight Benefits" has dire consequences that are here described as *zǎo shuāi* 早衰 "premature decrepitude." This term refers to a premature decline in one's physiological functions, before the natural aging

[4] For more information, see Donald Harper, *Early Chinese Medical Literature*, 428-432.

年五十，體重，耳目不聰明矣。
年六十，陰痿，氣大衰，九竅不利，下虛上實，涕泣俱出矣。
年四十而陰氣自半也，起居衰矣。

Nián sì shí ér yīn qì zì bàn yě,
qǐ jū shuāi yǐ.

Nián wǔ shí, tǐ zhòng,
ěr mù bù cōng míng yǐ.

Nián liù shí, yīn wěi, qì dà
shuāi, jiǔ qiào bù lì, xià xū
shàng shí, tì qì jù chū yǐ.

At the age of fifty, your body will become heavy and your ears and eyes lose their acuity!

At the age of sixty, your penis will wilt, your Qì will have greatly weakened, the nine orifices will not be freely passable, there will be vacuity below and repletion above, and discharge will flow from the eyes and nose.

This means that at the age of forty, your Yīn Qì will be halved on its own accord and your daily activities will weaken!

process as it is outlined in *Sù Wèn* Chapter 1, in multiples of seven for women and multiples of eight for men. Given the fact that the *Nèi Jīng* was literature that was written by and for men, the natural aging process, in contrast to the "premature decrepitude" described in later on this Section below, was conceived along the lines of the well-known passage from *Sù Wèn* Chapter 1 that is quoted above.

Concerning the halving of Yīn Qì and weakening of activities that Qí Bó describes as the consequence of this premature decrepitude, it makes obvious clinical sense that this phrase here points specifically to Kidney Essence and the prenatal Qì that is stored in the Kidney, which is said, in *Sù Wèn* Chapter *1*, to weaken at the age of five times eight in men. Here is Zhāng Zhìcōng's explanation:

Commentary by Zhāng Zhìcōng 張志聰

女子以七為紀，男子以八為紀。七損八益者，言陽常有余而陰常不足也。然陽氣生於陰精，知陰精之不足而無使其虧損，則二者可調。不知陰陽相生之道，而用此調養之法，則年未半百而早衰矣。男子以八為期，故四十而居半。陰氣，腎氣精氣也。陰氣漸虛，則起居倦矣。經曰：腎虛、肝虛、脾虛，皆令人體重煩寃。又曰：液脫者，骨肉屈伸不利。

Women take seven as their principle while men take eight as theirs. The Seven Decreases and Eight Increases refers to the fact that Yáng commonly has excess and Yīn commonly has insufficiency. This being so, Yáng Qì is engendered from Yīn Essence. Thus when we comprehend the insufficiency of Yīn Essence and do not allow it to get depleted, these two can be attuned. But when we do not comprehend the Way in which Yīn and Yáng mutually engender each other and the method for employing these to attune and nourish, we will suffer premature decrepitude before half our life is over! Men['s lives progress] in cycles of eight, and forty therefore means half their life. Yīn Qì is Kidney Qì and Essence Qì. When Yīn Qì becomes gradually vacuous, daily life becomes tiring. The Classic states: "Kidney vacuity, Liver vacuity, and Spleen vacuity, all of these cause the human body to become heavy, with vexation and distress." It also states: "Fluid desertion means that bending and stretching in the bones and flesh is inhibited."

* * *

LASTLY, A BRIEF NOTE IS IN ORDER CONCERNING THE PHRASE *YĪN WĚI* 陰痿, which literally means "Yīn wilts." It is certainly possible to read the expression here as such in a larger and more literal meaning. Nevertheless, in medical literature of even this early age, the technical meaning of this phrase as referring specifically to the wilting of the penis (frequently called *yīn jīng* 陰莖 "Yīn stalk" in sexual cultivation texts) and hence to a man's inability to maintain an erection during sexual intercourse, is well-established. Given that this whole passage is concerned with sexual cultivation, this is undoubtedly the meaning intended here. Moreover, because the orifices are not functioning properly, essence is exhausted in the lower body but the fluids pour out of the upper body in the form of uncontrollable discharge from the nose and eyes.

* * *

Commentary on Section Fourteen by Z'ev Rosenberg

MANY YEARS AGO I HAD TWO ALMOST IDENTICAL CASES OF YOUNG MEN IN their early to mid twenties, both recently graduated from university: The first individual was highly self-absorbed, young and handsome but obsessed with losing his hair. To this end, he took Propecia, a prostate drug, also used to prevent hair loss. His major complaint was "not being able to satisfy my girlfriend" due to unsatisfying erections, and an inability to perform sex more than once or twice a week. His pulse was large and scallion-stalk like, a bit soggy, and his tongue a light red color. I warmed his abdominal and lower back *shu* points with moxa, needled the Shàoyīn channel, and prescribed Guìzhī Jiā Lónggǔ Mǔlì Tāng 桂枝加龍骨牡蠣湯, which is perfect for this situation. He did not improve as rapidly as he would have liked, so I asked him if he masturbated, being clued by his pulse to loss of *jīng* Essence. He said he masturbated several times a day! On top of this fact, Propecia often has the side effect of weakening libido and ejaculation. Improvement began as he limited his sexual activity more to being with his girlfriend.

The second individual was also a handsome young man in his mid twenties, a graduate from university who was now in an acupuncture college. His main issues were extreme exhaustion after ejaculation, difficulties with sleep, and occasional palpitations. His tongue was light red and his pulse large and scallion-stalk like. He had had major problems with recreational drugs in college, which had depleted his *jīng* Essence. I also prescribed for him Guìzhī Jiā Lónggǔ Mǔlì Tāng, later on progressing to Shèn Qì Wán 腎氣丸 to supplement his kidneys. Improvement was slow but steady....

"If patients suffering from seminal loss present with stringlike tension in the lesser abdomen, yīn-head (penis) cold, dizzy vision, hair loss, and a pulse that is extremely vacuous, scallion-stalk, and slow, this means clear-grain (diarrhea with undigested food particles) blood collapse, and seminal loss. Whenever you see a pulse that is scallion-stalk and stirring or faint and tight, this means seminal loss in men and dreaming of intercourse in women. Cinnamon Twig Decoction Plus Dragon Bone and Oyster Shell (*guì zhī jiā lóng gǔ mǔ lì tāng* 桂枝加龍骨牡蠣湯) governs." (*Jīn Guì Yào Lüè* 金匱要略, Chapter 6)[5]

- CINNAMON TWIG (桂枝 guìzhī, Cinnamomi Ramulus) 3 liǎng
- PEONY ROOT (芍藥 sháoyào) 3 liǎng
- FRESH GINGER (生薑 shēngjiāng, Zingiberis Rhizoma Recens) 3 liǎng
- LICORICE (甘草 gāncǎo, Glycyrrhizae Radix) 2 liǎng
- JUJUBE (大棗 dàzǎo, Jujubae Fructus) 12 fruits
- DRAGON BONE (龍骨 lónggǔ, Mastodi Ossis Fossilia) 3 liǎng
- OYSTER SHELL (牡蠣 mǔlì, Ostreae Concha) 3 liǎng

[5] Wiseman and Wilms, *Jīn Guì Yào Lüè*, 133-134.

Section Fifteen

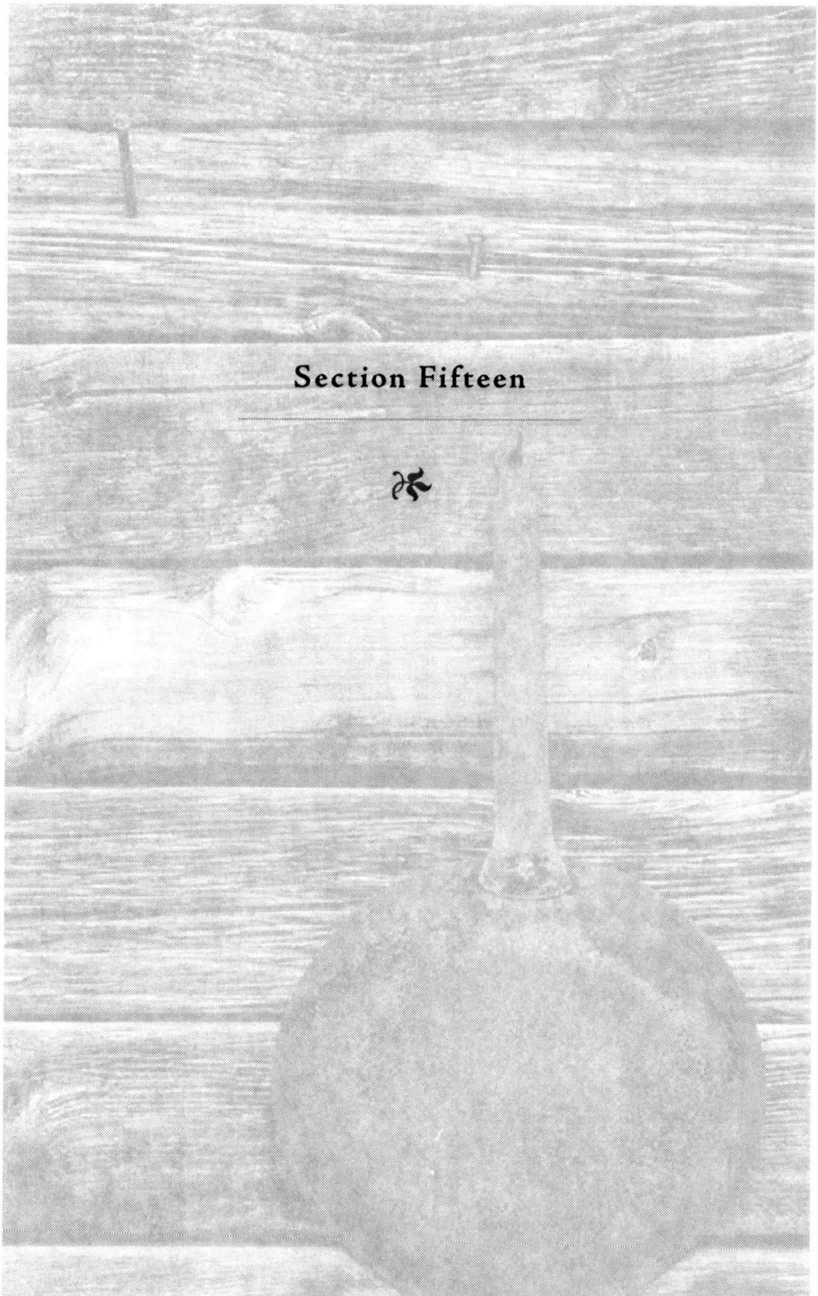

故曰：知之則強，不知則老。

故同出而名異耳。

智者察同，愚者察異；愚者不足，智者有餘。

Gù yuē: Zhī zhī zé qiáng,
bù zhī zé lǎo.

Gù tóng chū ér míng yì ěr.

Zhì zhě chá tóng, yú zhě chá yì;
yú zhě bù zú, zhì zhě yǒu yú.

Therefore I say: To know them results in vigor, and not to know them results in aging.

As such, they 'emerge from the same place and yet are different in name'.

Wise people investigate the commonalties; fools investigate the differences. Fools [are marked by] insufficiency; the wise by having excess.

THIS SECTION CONTINUES QÍ BÓ'S INSISTENCE THAT KNOWLedge of Yīn and Yáng and the methods for attuning them are the key to longevity and health. My literal translation of the phrase *zhī zhī* 知之 as "to know them" faithfully maintains the structure of the original text, which leaves the object of this knowing undefined. For the sake of readability in English, I had originally been tempted to interpret the object pronoun *zhī* 之 as "these rules for sexual intercourse" or as the above-mentioned "Seven Detriments and Eight Benefits." Nevertheless, in light of the following line, the word "them" is more likely to refer broadly to "Yīn and Yáng" in general. This interpretation is supported by the fact that this section is still part of Qí Bó's response to the Yellow Emperor's question about attuning Yīn and Yáng. Reading this line and the preceding section of the text only as referring to sexual cultivation, Zhāng Zhìcōng explains the first sentence in this way:

Commentary by Zhāng Zhìcōng 張志聰

知七損八益而能固守其精。則陰陽俱盛而筋骨壯強。
不知陰陽所生之原，以欲竭其精，以耗散其真，至半百而衰老矣。

When people know the Seven Detriments and Eight Benefits, they are able to secure and safeguard their Essence. As a result, Yīn and Yáng are both exuberant and the sinews and bones are firm and strong. When they do not know the source for the engenderment of Yīn and Yáng, they exhaust their Essence through their desires and scatter what is genuine through squandering. Thus they reach half of a hundred and are already weakened by old age!

IT IS IMPORTANT TO RECOGNIZE THE CENTRALITY OF SEXUAL CULTIvation as an effective technique for "nurturing life" (*yǎng shēng* 養生) in the theories and practices of the literate elite in early and medieval

有餘則耳目聰明，身體輕強，老者複壯，壯者益治。

是以聖人為無為之事，樂恬憺之能，從欲快志于虛無之守，故壽命無窮，與天地終，此聖人之治身也。

Yǒu yú zé ěr mù cōng míng,
shēn tǐ qīng qiáng, lǎo zhě fù zhuàng,
zhuàng zhě yì zhì.

Shì yǐ shèng rén wéi wú wèi zhī shì,
lè tián dàn zhī néng, cóng yù kuài
zhì yú xū wú zhī shǒu, gù shòu
mìng wú qióng, yù tiān dì zhōng,
cǐ shèng rén zhī zhì shēn yě.

For those who have excess, the ears and eyes have acuity and the body is light and vigorous. [As a result,] those who are [already] in their old age can return to their vigorous years and those who are [still] in their vigorous years can increase their management [of the body].

For this reason, the sages get things done by engaging in 'non-engagement,' take pleasure in their ability to maintain tranquillity and ease, follow their desires and joyfully direct their will to the safeguarding of emptiness and void. Therefore, their longevity is without bounds and joins Heaven and Earth to the end. This is the way in which the sages manage their bodies.

China. And if we are to treat this text strictly in its historical context and for historical accuracy, given our knowledge of early Hàn medical thought since the discovery of the Mǎwángduī and other contemporaneous manuscripts, this is the most faithful and honest reading of this passage. Sexual cultivation is certainly a core area of classical Chinese medicine that is, for historical and cultural reasons, largely ignored by contemporary practitioners, teachers, and students, both in Asia and the West. We can benefit from the information in the present passage in two ways: On the one hand, we can open our minds, trust and embrace the wisdom of the ancient sages, and start paying attention to the potential benefits and risks of sexual cultivation. The knowledge on this topic that is found in the medical classics can contribute to very real improvements in clinical practice, in terms of diagnosis, etiology, and treatment, along the lines suggested by Qí Bó here. Nevertheless, most modern practitioners will not want to change their medical practice (and prevailing cultural norms around sex) and risk making many patients uncomfortable with strange personal questions about their sex life. Instead, we can also read this entire discussion about attuning Yīn and Yáng in a more general sense as referring to diet, lifestyle, exercise, and climate, as well as to the equilibrium of Yīn and Yáng in the body, in terms of Blood and Qì, Heart and Kidney, upper and lower body, Fire and Water, and similar dualities.

Moving on to the second sentence, Qí Bó's statement that "they emerge from the same place and yet are different in name" has caused some disagreement among commentators. I have therefore translated it very literally, without writing my own interpretation into it. Discerning readers are welcome to create their own understanding of this statement and its function in the present context. It is, however, impossible to appreciate it fully without knowing that the famous five-character phrase is originally found in the beginning section of the *Dào Dé Jīng* 《道德經》 (Classic of the Way and Virtue-Power). I quote that passage in full here to show the intention of the original source text, which any of the early Hàn authors and readers of the *Nèi Jīng* would most certainly have recognized instantly.

Quotation from Láozi 老子[1]

道可道，非常道。名可名，非常名。

無名天地之始；有名萬物之母。

故常無欲，以觀其妙；常有欲，以觀其徼。

此兩者，同出而異名，同謂之玄。玄之又玄，衆妙之門。

The Dào that can be taken as a Dào is not the Dào that endures. The name that can be used as a name is not the name that endures.

That which has no name is the beginning of Heaven and Earth; that which has a name is the mother of the Myriad Things.

Hence enduring absence of wants allows us to observe the subliminal; enduring presence of wants allows us to observe the perimeter.

These two! They share the same origin yet differ in name. Their sameness is what we call "obscure." Further obscured in this obscurity, the gateway to everything that is subliminal!

THE QĪNG DYNASTY COMMENTATOR GĀO SHÌZŌNG SUGGESTS A narrow reading of this phrase in the present context of *Sù Wèn* Chapter 5: He interprets it as referring to the fact that all humans share the same origin, namely the healthy potential of the newborn baby, but end up with opposite characteristics or "names," namely "vigor" 強 or "aging" 老, depending on the person's ability to attune

[1] *Dào Dé Jīng* 《道德經》 Section 1.

Yīn and Yáng and properly practice sexual intercourse. This certainly seems like a fitting interpretation in the specific context of the chapter.

* * *

Commentary by Gāo Shìzōng 高士宗

同出於斯世之中，而強老之名則異耳。

All people emerge into this age in the same way, and yet they differ in terms of the name 'vigor' and 'old age'.

* * *

COMPARED TO THIS, ZHĀNG ZHÌCŌNG'S READING IS MORE CLINICALLY oriented, contrasting the common origin, still interpreted as birth by both authors, in Yīn Essence, but different names in later manifestation as *Shén*, Qì, and Essence.

* * *

Commentary by Zhang Zhicong 張志聰

『同出而名異』：神氣生於陰精，故同出於天乙之真，而有精氣神三者之異名耳。

"Emerge from the same place and yet are different in name": Because the Shén and Qì are engendered in Yīn Essence, they emerge from the same place in genuineness of tiān yǐ, and yet they have the three different names of jīng (Essence), Qì, and Shén.

* * *

THE MAIN POINT TO TAKE AWAY HERE IS PERHAPS THAT QÍ BÓ IS emphasizing the common origin of all humans, their identical potential, at birth, to live out their heavenly allotted lifespan along the lines of physical development and aging that are described in *Sù Wèn* Chapter 1 in multiples of seven for women and eight for men. It is only when we are ignorant of attuning Yīn and Yáng and therefore disturb our physiological equilibrium, whether by squandering essence, by indulging in emotional outbursts, through improper diet, or by failing to align with the changes of Yīn and Yáng in the external environment, that our bodies age and decline in vigor before their proper time.

While the clinical interpretation suggested by Zhāng above appears reasonable and medically meaningful, the following line, however, that 'Those who are wise investigate what is the same; fools investigate what is different," suggests that we dig a little deeper. Here we may want to recall the critique of human language, artifice, and dualistic thinking expressed most prominently by *Zhuāngzi* in numerous passages and stories, from the frog in the well to the happiness of the fish and "three in the morning."

* * *

Quotation from Zhuāngzi 莊子[2]

至人無己，神人無功，聖人無名。

The accomplished person is without a self. The spirit person is without effort. The sage is without a name.

* * *

[2] *Zhuāngzi* 《莊子》 Chapter 1, *Xiāo Yáo Yóu* 逍遙遊 (Free and Footloose Roaming).

This statement that "Those who are wise investigate what is the same; fools investigate what is different" in combination with the previous line shows where the authors of the *Nèi Jīng* place their emphasis. But how are we to interpret and apply this guideline in clinical practice? By now, it has become clear that what the text is referring to as "same in origin" (*tóng chū* 同出), which is the stated goal of what wise people should investigate, must somehow refer to our common source in an equilibrium of Yīn and Yáng, the unity that lies beyond all dualistic manifestations, or, in the medical context, our original state of health and longevity. Likewise, where humans differ from each other is in the way in which the physiological processes of maturing and aging play out, with the result that some of us age more quickly than others. Nevertheless, the first thing any physician must do when diagnosing a patient is to figure out where the patient's specific state at the moment differs from the norm, where things have gone awry, or in other words, precisely this difference between health and sickness. How are we to restore equilibrium without first knowing where it is disturbed? My best answer is that this part of the *Great Discourse* does not give medical advice to the physician in charge of treating others but to the elite readers who were interested in cultivating their own health. From this perspective, wise people focus their study and attention on maintaining the equilibrium in perfect health and hence "have excess," especially when they are wise enough to pay attention to sexual cultivation, preserving Essence, avoiding overexertion and emotional upsets, and harmonizing Yīn and Yáng when they are still in their prime. Fools, on the other hand, are marked by ignorance and therefore squander their health recklessly until it is too late and they are plagued by irreversible insufficiency.

The last two lines of this section describe the benefits of following a wise lifestyle in language that is strikingly similar to the first two paragraphs of *Sù Wèn* Chapter 1. In addition, both passages are clearly influenced by the ideals and language found in Daoist philosophical literature.

Quotations from Láozi 老子[3]

天下皆知美之為美，斯惡已。皆知善之為善，斯不善已。

故有無相生，難易相成，長短相較，高下相傾，音聲相和，前後相隨。

是以聖人處無為之事，行不言之教；萬物作焉而不辭，生而不有，為而不恃，功成而弗居。夫唯弗居，是以不去。

The awareness in all Under Heaven of the "beauty" of the beautiful thereby causes the existence of "ugly." The awareness of the "goodness" of the good thereby causes the existence of "not good."

Thus being and non-being engender one another; difficult and easy co-create one another; long and short exist in comparison with one another; high and low lean on one another; music and sound harmonize with one another; and before and after follow upon one another.

For this reason the sages involve themselves in affairs of non-engagement and enact teachings of no-speaking. With regard to the Myriad Things, they create them by this but do not leave them behind, engender them but do not possess them, engage with them but do not depend on them, accomplish in deeds, but do not dwell on them. It is only by not dwelling on them that they do not lose them.

[3] Láozi 老子 *Dào Dé Jīng* 《道德經》 Sections 2 and 3.

不尚賢，使民不爭；不貴難得之貨， 使民不為盜；不見可欲，使心不亂。

是以聖人之治，虛其心，實其腹，弱其志，強其骨。

常使民無知無欲，使夫知者不敢為也。

為無為，則無不治。

Not placing worthies above everybody else keeps the common people from arguing. Not valuing goods that are difficult to obtain keeps the common people from becoming thieves. Not putting desirable things on display keeps their hearts from being disordered.

For this reason the sages govern by emptying the common people's hearts and filling their bellies, by weakening their wills and strengthening their bones.

They constantly make the common people be without knowledge and without wants and make those who know not dare to act on account of that.

By engaging in non-engagement, there is nothing that is not put in good order.

* * *

At the same time, however, we should also recognize the reference to Confucius' *Lùn Yǔ* 《論語》 (Analects) in the phrase 從欲 "follow their desires."

Quotation from Confucius[4]

子曰：吾十有五而志于學、三十而立、四十而不惑、五十而知天命、六十而耳順、七十而從心所欲、不踰矩。

The Master said: 'At fifteen, I had set my mind on studying; at thirty, I had established myself; at forty, I was no longer confused; at fifty, I knew the Mandate of Heaven; at sixty, my ears were compliant; at seventy, I was able to follow my Heart's desires without transgressing the rules.

[4] Confucius 孔子 *Lùn Yǔ* 《論語》 Book 2, *Wéi Zhèng* 為政 (Enacting Government).

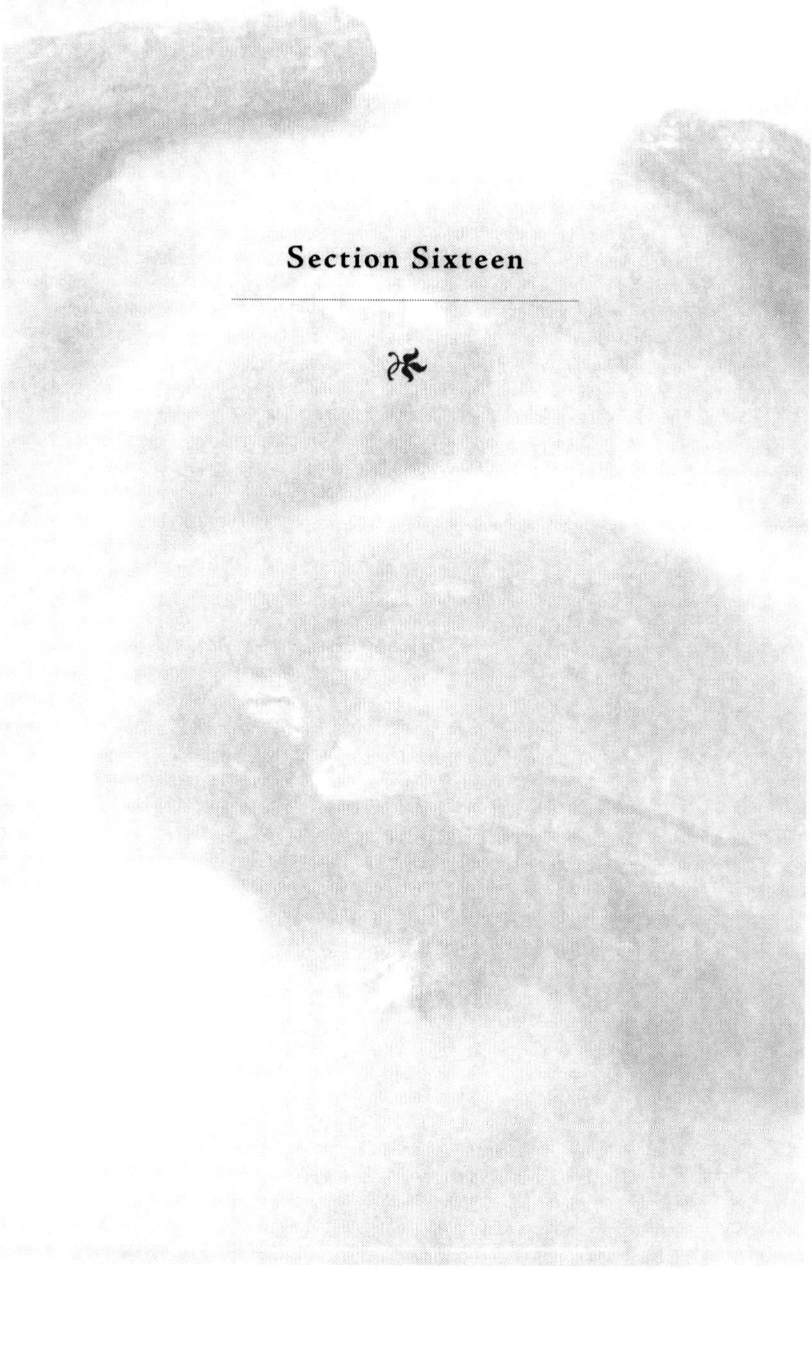

Section Sixteen

天不足西北，故西北方陰也，而人右耳目不如左明也。
地不滿東南，故東南方陽也，而人左手足不如右強也。

Tiān bù zú xī běi,
gù xī běi fāng yīn yě,
ér rén yòu ěr mù bù
rú zuǒ míng yě.
Dì bù mǎn dōng nán,
gù dōng nán fāng yáng yě,
ér rén zuǒ shǒu zú bù
rú yòu qiáng yě.

The insufficiency of Heaven in the northwest is the reason why the northwestern direction is Yīn and why in humans the right ear and eye are not as perceptive as the left. The failure of Earth to fill up the southeast is the reason why the southeastern direction is Yáng, and why in humans the left hand and foot are not as strong as the right ones."

Commentary by Wáng Bīng 王冰

在上故法天，在下故法地。夫陰陽之應天地，猶水之在器也，器圓則水圓，器曲則水曲，人之血氣亦如是，故隨不足則邪氣留居之。

Above, we thus conform to Heaven, and below, we conform to Earth. Now the way in which Yīn and Yáng resonate in Heaven and Earth is just like water inside a container. If the container is round, the water is also round. If the container is curved, the water is also curved. A person's Blood and Qì are also like this. Thus in accordance with any insufficiency, evil Qì will take up residence there.

WÁNG BĪNG'S COMMENTARY ON THIS SECTION MAKES PERfect sense and reiterates the direct resonances between Yīn-Yáng in the macrocosm and in the human body.

Employing simple direct reasoning, Wáng Bīng points out that any time there is a vacuum anywhere in the body, evil Qì will take advantage of this defect and fill it, just like water filling up all the nooks and crannies in dry soil, or insects or wind finding a path into an old home that has cracks in the walls.

We can easily visualize the association of east with left and west with right when we remember that traditionally the ruler, or the cartographer, is positioned up in the north, facing south. It may also help to remember that the sun, associated with Yáng, rises in the east but sets in the west, and that the northwestern region of China is known to be much colder than the southeast. While the above passage may strike the clinically oriented reader as somewhat odd and perhaps not immediately useful in medical application, its function in this chapter is not to provide clinical advice. Instead, it is meant here to reiterate from yet another angle the direct correlation—one may even say identity—between the body of the sage and the macrocosmic

帝曰：何以然？

岐伯曰：東方陽也，陽者其精並於上，並於上則上明而下虛，故使耳目聰明而手足不便也。西方陰也。陰者其精並於下，並於下則下盛而上虛，故其耳目不聰明而手足便也。

Dì yuē: Hé yǐ rán?

Qí Bó yuē: Dōng fāng yáng yě, yáng zhě qí jīng bìng yú shàng, bìng yú shàng zé shàng míng ér xià xū, gù shǐ ěr mù cōng míng ér shǒu zú bù biàn yě. Xī fāng yīn yě. Yīn zhě qí jīng bìng yú xià, bìng yú xià zé xià shèng ér shàng xū, gù qí ěr mù bù cōng míng ér shǒu zú biàn yě.

The Emperor asked: "Why is that so?"

Qí Bó answered: **"The eastern direction indeed is Yáng. As for Yáng, its Essence gathers in the upper body. Because it gathers in the upper body, the upper body is bright and the lower body is vacuous. Hence this causes the ears and eyes to be perceptive while the hands and feet do not move with ease. The western direction is Yīn. As for Yīn, its Essence gathers in the lower body. Because it gathers in the lower body, the lower body is abundant and the upper body is vacuous. Hence such a person's ears and eyes are not perceptive but the hands and feet move with ease.**

body of the universe. What is true in the cardinal directions of the universe also holds true for any human body that has managed to align itself in perfect harmony with the universal changes inherent in the Dào. And that is the reason why the sage, as one who is able to avoid providing opportunities for evil Qì to sneak in and take up residence in the body, is able to live forever, until the end of the lifespan of Heaven and Earth.

This identification between the sage's body and the macrocosmic body has been taken literally by countless practitioners and scholars of Chinese medicine through the centuries. Gāo Shìzōng's commentary of this line expresses this sentiment:

* * *

Commentary by Gāo Shìzōng 高士宗

聖人壽命與天地終，則人之形體即天地之形體也。

The sage's longevity comes to an end together with Heaven and Earth. This means then that the human body is identical with the body of Heaven and Earth.

* * *

The ears and eyes are located in the head, which is associated with Heaven, Yáng, roundness, and clear Qì rising. As such, an imbalance of Qì marked by abundance in the upper body and insufficiency in the lower body manifests in improved function in the sense organs of the head but impaired function in the "hands and feet," which refers to the four limbs, here standing for the lower body, which is associated with Earth, Yīn, squareness, and turbid Qì descending. Similarly, abundance in the lower body and insufficiency in the upper body manifests with a smooth operation of the four limbs but a lack of perceptivity in the sense organs of the head.

One difficulty with this passage is that it appears to contradict other passages where *jīng* Essence is associated with Earth and the

故俱感于邪，其在上則右甚，在下則左甚。
此天地陰陽所不能全也，故邪居之。

Gù jù gǎn yú xié,
qí zài shàng zé yòu shèn,
zài xià zé zuǒ shèn.
Cǐ tiān dì yīn yáng suǒ
bù néng quán yě,
gù xié jū zhī.

For this reason,
whenever there is a
contraction of evil,
it is worse on the right
if it is in the upper body,
while it is worse on the left
if it is in the lower body.
These are the locations
where Heaven and Earth
and Yīn and Yáng
are unable to be complete.
For this reason,
evil takes up residence there.

lower body, while Qì is associated with the upper body and Heaven. Here, however, the text mentions both Yáng Essence and Yīn Essence, and associates Yáng Essence with the upper body. To resolve this apparent conundrum, it may help to interpret "Yáng Essence" and "Yīn Essence" here as two kinds of Qì, associated with Yáng and Yīn respectively.

As so often in the *Nèi Jīng* and in this chapter, there are increasingly deeper levels at which we can sub-divide a simple apparent Yīn-Yáng duality between such clear opposites as Flavor 味 and Qì 氣, to name an example from Section 2 above, into further subdivisions of Yīn and Yáng in each of these polarities. Thus, while Flavor is described there as Yīn in contrast to the Yáng nature of Qì, it is later in Section 3 further differentiated into concentrated Flavor, associated with Yīn within Yīn, and diluted Flavor, which is Yáng within Yīn. Similarly, we may start out with a polarity between Qì, associated with Heaven and the upper body, and Essence, associated with Earth and the lower body. In the passage here, though, we now encounter a Yáng Essence, associated with Heaven, and a Yīn Essence, associated with Earth. Going even a step further, Zhāng Zhìcōng in his commentary equates Essence with Heaven, and Form with Earth, an idea that we will encounter again in the following section of the *Great Treatise*, but then distinguishes between Yáng Essence and Yīn Essence:

* * *

Commentary by Zhāng Zhìcōng 張志聰

天有精，地有形。東方陽也。其精氣上升而並於上，
並於上則上盛而下虛。故使人之耳目聰明而手足不便也。
西方陰也。其精氣下降而並於下，並於下則下盛而上虛。
故其人之耳目不聰明而手足便也。此以天地之左右而言也。

Heaven has Essence; Earth has Form. The eastern direction is Yáng. Its Essence Qì rises up and gathers in the upper body. Gathering in the upper body, it makes the upper body exuberant and the lower body vacuous. Therefore it causes the person's eyes and ears to be perceptive but the hands and feet to not move with ease. The western direction is Yīn. Its Essence Qì descends and gathers in the lower body. Gathering in the lower body, it makes the lower body exuberant and the upper body vacuous. Therefore such a person's ears and eyes are not perceptive but the hands and feet move with ease. This line is speaking about the left and right side of Heaven and Earth.

* * *

Rather than making yet another futile attempt at resolving through logical gymnastics what appears as a rational contradiction within the narrow confines of human language, we are better off once again to embrace the fact that reality can look one way from one perspective and look completely different from another perspective. It is one of the great strenths and beauties of traditional Chinese medicine that it offers the experienced practitioner any number of perspectives from which to approach a situation at any given moment, with vastly different answers and outcomes based on the chosen path. But it is also this characteristic that makes it so difficult and confusing for beginning students of this medicine, especially ones who comes from a scientific background where reality is either white or black, this or that, cat or dog, right or wrong. Chinese philosophers have been discussing this conundrum ever since the famous discourse by Gongsun Long 公孫龍 on a white horse not being a horse (*bái mǎ fēi mǎ* 白馬非馬) around 300 BCE. In the present case, the point of this passage is to offer additional evidence for the central premise of this chapter, namely the clear and unequivocal resonance between the macrocosm (as Heaven and Earth) and the human body (as in the sense organs in the head and the limbs in the lower body) through the paradigm of Yīn and Yáng. This passage here offers just one more concrete evidence and illustration for how this resonance manifests in concrete terms.

Section Seventeen

故天有精，地有形；天有八紀，地有五里，故能為萬物之父母。

清陽上天，濁陰歸地，是故天地之動靜，神明為之綱紀，

故能以生長收藏，終而複始。

Gù tiān yǒu jīng, dì yǒu xíng;
tiān yǒu bā jì, dì yǒu wǔ lǐ,
gù néng wéi wàn wù zhī fù mǔ.

Qīng yáng shàng tiān, zhuó yīn guī dì,
shì gù tiān dì zhī dòng jìng,
shén míng wéi zhī gāng jì,
gù néng yǐ shēng zhǎng shōu cáng,
zhōng ér fù shǐ.

Therefore, Heaven has Essence
and Earth has Form;
Heaven has the Eight Threads
and Earth has the Five Patterns.
As such, they are able to serve
as father and mother
of the Myriad Things.

Clear Yáng rises to Heaven,
turbid Yīn homes to the Earth.
As such, concerning the activity and
stillness of Heaven and Earth,
the shén míng takes these as its
'lead ropes and connecting strands'
and is therefore able, by means of
sprouting, growth, harvest, and
storage, to bring [the myriad things]
to an end and start [them] anew.

SECTION SEVENTEEN FIRST OUTLINES HOW HEAVEN AND EARTH relate to Yīn and Yáng to fuel the cycle of life and then delves into additional manifestations of concrete resonances between changes in the macrocosm and in the microcosm, in terms of Yīn-Yáng and Five-Agent correlations but also in terms of climatic factors and other apparently random associations. These do not follow the schematic patterns that we are used to from other chapters or the earlier sections in the *Great Discourse* but instead seem to express a genuine desire to map the distinguishing features of the external world onto the internal landscape of the human body on the basis of clinical experience. As such, this section first returns to the dyad of Heaven and Earth, and the associated forces of Yáng and Yīn, and then introduces how this dyad turns into a triad, with the addition of humanity in the middle as one of the locations where the cosmic forces of Heaven and Earth meet and become manifest.

I am struck by the similarity between this perspective and one I encountered recently in a book titled *Braiding Sweetgrass* by Native American scientist Robin Wall Kimmerer that attempts to answer questions of nature with the tools of science as well as the guidance of indigenous teachings. She describes the instructions by the traditional Potawatomi basket maker John Pigeon in the process of assembling the bottom of a hand-woven basket made from Black Ash splints by laying out four strips in a symmetrical cross:

> Our people honor the four sacred directions and the powers resident there. Where the two basket strips meet, at the intersection of those four directions, is right were we stand as humans, trying to find balance among them...Once the eight spokes of the framework are twined into place with the thinnest possible strips, each basket begins to grow....
>
> In weaving well-being for land and people, we need to pay attention to the lessons of the three rows. Ecological well-being and the laws of nature are always the first row. Without them, there is no basket of plenty. Only if that first circle is in place can we

> weave the second. The second reveals material welfare, the subsistence of human needs. Economy built upon ecology. But with only two rows in place, the basket is still in jeopardy of pulling apart. It's only when the third row comes that the first two can hold together, Here is where ecology, economics, and spirit are woven together. By using materials as if they were a gift, and returning the gift through worthy use, we find balance. I think that third row goes by many names: Respect. Reciprocity. All our Relations. I think of it as the spirit row. Whatever the name, the three rows represent recognition that our lives depend on one another, human needs being only one row in the basket that must hold us all. In relationship, the separate splints become a whole basket, sturdy and resilient enough to carry us into the future.[1]

Regardless of how closely we may want to match each of Kimmerer's three rows of ecology, economics, and spirit with the Chinese traditional Three Powers (*sān cái* 三才) of Heaven, Humanity, and Earth (*tiān rén dì* 天人地), I have no doubt that the Yellow Emperor and his companions would have appreciated the notion of reciprocity, interdependence, and relationship between these three dimensions. It is the beauty of Chinese medicine, and also one of its greatest contributions to contemporary medicine and science, that it so eloquently reminds us of this need for reciprocity, humility, and gratitude for the world around us and its innumerable gifts. It explains clearly that as humans, it is not our role to rule over Heaven and Earth but to align and harmonize our internal and external actions with the cosmic forces in the interplay of Heaven and Earth, Yáng and Yīn, which are far greater than we are. From this perspective, the strength of the physician does not lie in correcting problems of misalignment between the cosmic body and the individual and social human body by changing the external environment, but by adapting the human body to the far greater and more powerful cosmic one. As such, the greatest virtue of the physician, or any human, is to possess *shén míng* 神明,

[1] Robin Wall Kimmerer, *Braiding Sweetgrass*, 152-3.

"spirit illumination," the ability to establish a connection between the human individual and Heaven through the *Shén*.

Looking at the above passage in the *Great Discourse* line by line, we encounter a number of expressions that require an explanation. Already in the first line, most commentators agree that the term *bā jì* 八紀, translated above as "Eight Threads," here refers to the eight seasonal divisions of the calendar year: the vernal and autumnal equinoxes *chūnfēn* 春分 / *qiūfēn* 秋分; summer and winter solstices *xiàzhì* 夏至 / *dōngzhì* 冬至, and the beginnings of the four seasons *lìchūn* 立春, *lìxià* 立夏, *lìqiū* 立秋, *lìdōng* 立冬. For this reason, later Chinese dictionaries and commentaries tend to cite this particular passage as proof for this interpretation. This explanation is most likely based on Wáng Bīng's explanation of the term as *bā jié* 八節 (eight seasonal nodes). Rather than limiting our understanding of the present passage to this meaning, I have chosen to translate it very literally so that you can make up your own mind on what this phrase may mean here. I would like to remind the reader of the use of this character in the first line of the chapter, in the famous statement: "As for Yīn and Yáng, they are the Dào of Heaven and Earth. They are the guide ropes and connecting threads of the Myriad Things." In that context, the character *jì* 紀 referred to the connecting strands of a net, usually interpreted as the more discernible, measurable aspects of the Myriad Things, as opposed to the grand universal principles represented by the term *gāng* 綱 "guide rope." In other contexts, especially in the compound *jīng jì* 經紀, the term refers to the weft (as in "warp and weft" of a woven piece of fabric).

Still in the first line, we then find the equally mysterious phrase *wǔ lǐ* 五里 (literally "five miles" or "five villages"), which I have translated as "five patterns": Different editions of this chapter write the character with different radicals as 里, 理, or even as 裡, reflecting their editors' interpretation. I read it as 理 (ordering principle, pattern, or underlying structure, originally the grain in jade, see my discussion above at the beginning of Section Six (page 151) because it is such a perfect contrast to the "Eight Threads." Most commentators define this expression in turn as the four cardinal directions and the center, in the sense of the modern *dàolǐ* 道理 (principle), but Wáng Bīng for one

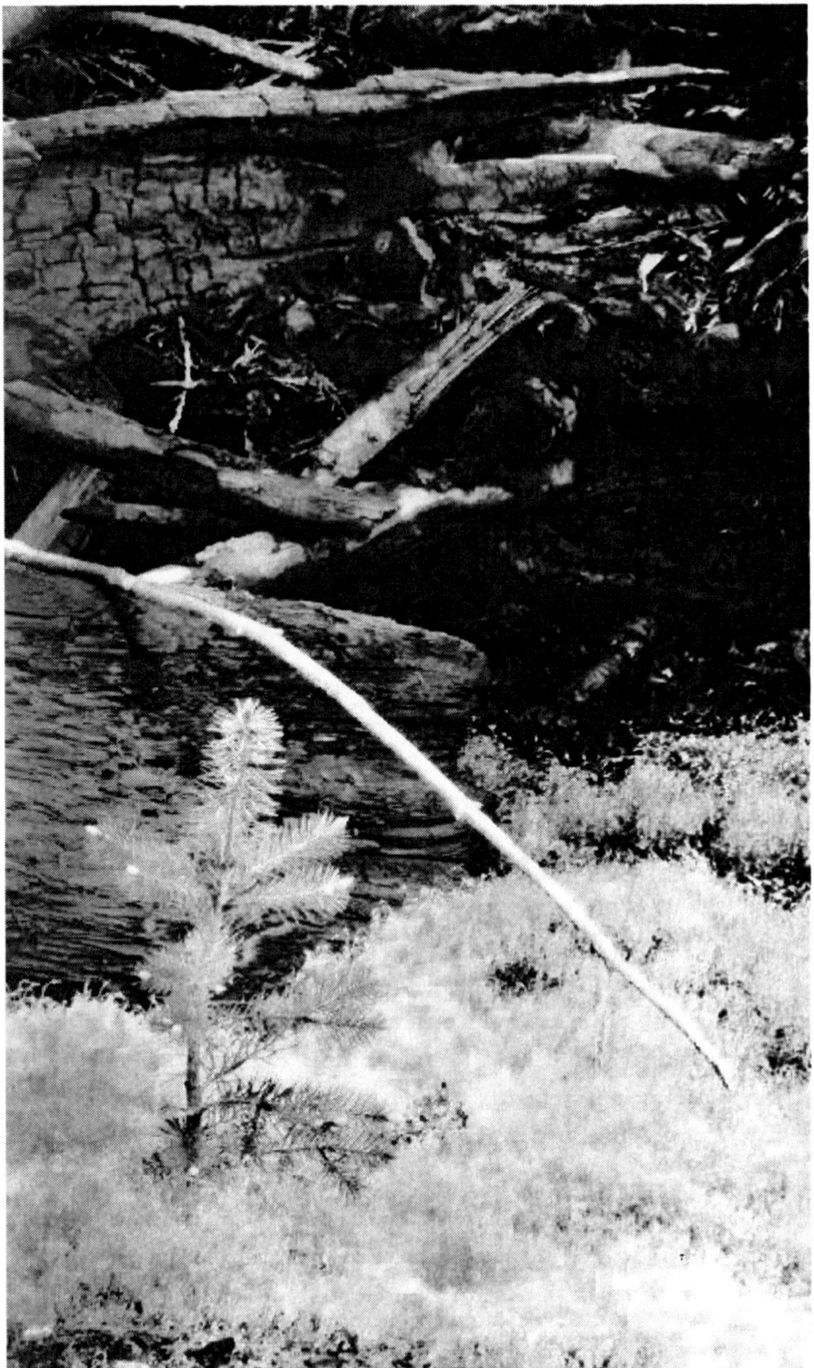

actually reads it as "village" (*lǐ* 里) in the sense of "neighborhoods." Zhāng Zhìcōng paraphrases the entire line in this way: "Heaven has the structural network of the Eight Directions. Earth has the structural principle of the Five Dynamic Agents" (天有八方之紀綱。地有五行之道理).

The second half of this first passage in Section Seventeen refers back to the introductory statement of the *Great Discourse* that Yīn and Yáng are the "palace of the *shén míng*." See my discussion of this passage there for leaving the term *shén míng* untranslated (see page 151). As Zhāng Zhìcōng explains in his commentary to the passage here, "the *shén míng* is what engenders the Five Qì and causes substantive change among the Five Dynamic Agents" (神明者，生五氣，化五行者也).

The text then goes on to reiterate that the root of all creation is found in this dynamic oscillation of Yīn and Yáng, based on their natural tendency to move apart and come back together, with clear Yáng rising up to Heaven and turbid Yīn sinking down to Earth and reversing direction when they reach their extreme. This movement is what makes the cycle of life possible, expressed here in the four characters *sheng* 生, *zhǎng* 長, *shōu* 收, *cáng* 藏 "birth, growth, harvest, and storage." Already mentioned in Section Five above, these terms are the actions or tendencies of seasonal Qì associated with each of the four seasons, as laid out in detail in *Sù Wèn* Chapter 2. The action associated with spring, 生 *shēng*, which is generally translated as "birth," can here also be translated more literally as "sprouting," based on the etymology of the character, an image of a plant sprouting out of the ground, and the agricultural connotation of these activities.

惟賢人上配天以養頭，下象地以養足，
中傍人事以養五臟。

Wéi xián rén shàng pèi tiān yǐ yǎng tóu,
xià xiàng dì yǐ yǎng zú,
zhōng bàng rén shì yǐ yǎng wǔ zàng.

It is only paragons of virtue
who [are able to] match up with
Heaven above and thereby
nourish the head,
imitate Earth below
and thereby nourish the feet,
and in the middle stay close
to human affairs and thereby
nourish the Five Zàng Organs.

THE LAST PART OF THIS SECTION INTRODUCES THE READER TO A WAY of being in the world that differs subtly from that of the sage (*shèng rén* 聖人), which we have encountered above in Section 15. There, we learned that "Sages get things done by engaging in non-engagement, take pleasure in their ability to maintain tranquility and ease, follow their desires, and joyfully direct their will to the safeguarding of emptiness and void. Therefore, their longevity is without bounds and joins Heaven and Earth to the end. This is the way in which the sages manage their bodies" (聖人為無為之事，樂恬憺之能，從欲快志于虛無之守，故壽命無窮，與天地終，此聖人之治身也。). In contrast, the present line describes the ideal behavior of a different kind of person: *xián rén* 賢人 or in my translation "paragon of virtue." Is it just a stylistic choice by the author to use a different character here to refer to a figure of exalted virtue and wisdom, or is this wording intentional and carries a set of associations that we need to be aware of? In other words, is there a difference between a sage and a paragon of virtue that the sensitive reader needs to grasp, which can help us shed light on this line here?

Most directly, we can try to fit these two terms, as is often done, into the strait jacket of the two traditional main branches of classical Chinese philosophy by dusting off that convenient old opposition: On the one hand we have Daoism, concerned with individual cultivation outside the norms and restraints of human relations, with grasping the cosmic and ultimately ineffable Dào, and with finding and restoring harmony and One-ness with the natural realm for the purpose of longevity and immortality. These ideals are represented by the concepts of the sage (*shèng rén* 聖人), and in a state even more advanced and further removed from ordinary human existence, the "perfected person" (*zhén rén* 真人). Confucianism, on the other hand, humbly concentrates on ordering human relations, beginning with the individual in their closest family relationships and extending all the way to governing an empire, by studying and practicing the Way of the ancients and cultivating basic human virtues like respect, integrity, compassion, and justice. The ideal person in this context is usually referred to as the paragon of virtue (*xián rén* 賢人). Following the description in the line above, this ideal figure "in the middle stays close to human affairs."

As will become apparent shortly, though, this standard dualistic opposition between "Daoism" and "Confucianism," which was introduced first for bibliographic purposes in the Hàn dynasty many centuries after the composition of the classical philosophical literature, does not make much sense in the context of medical literature of the Hàn or later periods. In fact, I would argue that we are better off studying each classical philosopher on his own and then contemplating how each of them contributed to the powerful creative synthesis that culminated in the composition of the *Nèi Jīng*. Trying to view the "Daoist" and "Confucian" influences in Hàn dynasty medical literature as two distinct strands that can be studied separately and were supposedly promoted by followers of two distinct philosophical schools, resulting in distinct traditions of medical theory and practice, quickly leads to a dead end. Instead, I suggest that we approach classical Chinese medicine as a strong braid, consisting of numerous inseparable strands of philosophy, cosmology, religion, science, shamanism, folk knowledge of medicinal substances and physical manipulation, and increasingly also elite literati medical expertise. In my experience, disentangling this braid and separating the strands tends to lead to disintegration and to the unintended loss of important aspects, without which the remaining strands no longer make sense as an internally coherent system. Like most other teachers of this subject, I too continue to employ the questionable terms "Daoist" or "Confucian" at times as shortcuts for ease of communication to point my audience in a certain general direction. The present passage, however, is the perfect example for the dangers and limitations of this approach:

As mentioned in the line discussed here, "It is only paragons of virtue who [are able to] match up with Heaven above and thereby nourish the head, imitate Earth below and thereby nourish the feet, and in the middle stay close to human affairs and thereby nourish the Five *Zàng* Organs." To shed light on the meaning of these ideal paragons of virtue, and perhaps tease out a contrast to the sages we have encountered in Section 15 above, here is an excerpt from the very end of *Sù Wèn* Chapter 1 that introduces two additional, even more advanced types of ideal humans, namely the "Perfected Person" (*zhēn rén* 真人) and the "accomplished person" (*zhì rén* 至人). Given that we are mostly dealing with the lower levels of cultivation and accomplishment in the present book and that the two highest levels are described as having existed in what was already the ancient and middle past during the Yellow Emperor's time, I choose to ignore these first two categories in my discussion below.

* * *

Quotation from Sù Wèn[2]

黄帝曰：余聞上古有真人者，提挈天地，把握陰陽，呼吸精氣，獨立守神，肌肉若一，故能壽敝天地，無有終時。此其道生。

中古之時，有至人者，淳德全道，和於陰陽，調於四時，去世離俗，積精全神，游行天地之間，視聽八達之外。此蓋益其壽命而強者也，亦歸於真人。

其次有聖人者，處天地之和，從八風之理；適嗜欲於世俗之間，無恚嗔之心，行不欲離於世，被服章，舉不欲觀於俗，外不勞形於事，內無思想之患，以恬愉為務，以自得為功，形體不敝，精神不散，亦可以百數。

其次有賢人者，法則天地，象似日月，辯列星辰，逆從陰陽，分別四時，將從上古，合同於道，亦可使益壽而有極時。

The Yellow Emperor said: "I have heard that in the ancient past there were perfected persons. These people held up Heaven and Earth, were able to play with Yīn and Yáng, inhaled and exhaled Essence and Qì, stood upright on their own and kept their Spirit well-guarded, and had a body that was as if unified. Therefore they were able to live so long as to wear Heaven and Earth ragged, without a time of ending. This was their life in the Dào.

[2] *Sù Wèn* 《素問》 Chapter 1.

In the more recent past, there were accomplished persons. Their Virtue-Power undiluted and their Dào intact, they were in harmony with Yīn and Yáng and attuned to the Four Seasons. Having left behind the world of ordinary mortals, they collected Essence and kept their Spirit complete, traveled freely in the space between Heaven and Earth, and were able to see and hear beyond the far reaches of the Eight Directions. This, then, was how they must have increased their lifespan and become strong. [In that case?], they can also be counted among the perfected people.

On a lower level after these there are the sages, who reside in harmony with Heaven and Earth and follow the ordering principle of the Eight Winds. Adapting their preferences and desires to life among the common people, they carry no grudges or anger in their heart. In their actions, they do not want to distance themselves from the world, and in the clothing and adornments they wear, as well as in their activities, they do not want to be looked up to by the common people. On the outside, they do not tax their Form in their work, and on the inside, they do not trouble themselves with preoccupied thinking. They handle their responsibilities with calm contentment and achieve results with self-satisfaction. Their trunk and limbs do not get worn out, their Essence Spirit does not get scattered, and hence they are thereby also able to live for a hundred years.

Lower than these again are the paragons of virtue. Conforming to Heaven and Earth, imitating the role of the sun and the moon, they differentiate and arrange in order the stars and heavenly time markers, greet the arrival and follow the departure of Yīn and Yáng, and distinguish between the Four Seasons. Wanting to follow [the example of the perfected persons in] Remote Antiquity, they are in complete unity and accord with the Dào and are thereby also able to increase their lifespan and yet their lifetime has a limit.

* * *

In the standard interpretation of this important passage, the first half of this quotation describes the Daoist ideal of transcending the limitations of the physical Form in human existence and of connecting with Heaven and merging with Heaven's Qì to live forever, while the second half describes the Confucian goal of becoming an ethical human being through the cultivation of Virtue along the lines of the *Dà Xué* 《大學》 (Great Learning). While continuing to actively participate in society, these advanced humans are able to live out their heavenly allotted lifespan instead of ending their lives prematurely as the result of overexertion, careless scattering of Essence, and loss of safeguarding of the *shén*. In contrast to these sages and paragons of virtue, ordinary humans shorten their lives as the result of carelessness and exposure to external evils or internal overindulgence in sexual intercourse, dietary irregularities, or emotional extremes. Here we see that in this passage, at least in the lowest two tiers, the ordinary division between "Daoists" and "Confucians" does not make sense since both the sages and the paragons of virtue are characterized by active skillful involvement in the human realm as well as by longevity due to their ability to live in harmony with the macrocosm. The difference between these two, at least in this quote, appears to be one merely of degree of cultivation, not direction of their effort towards engagement with either society or with the natural environment. One possible explanation for this conundrum may be that we modern humans might see and experience a separation between the human realm and the macrocosm, both in its Earthly expression as ecology and in its Heavenly expression as spirit, if you want to stay with Kimmerer's three rows of basket weaving. And this division, which is unfortunately for too many of us a reality of our lived experience in modern society and culture to the point where we experience "species loneliness," then manifests in the standard explanations of Chinese philosophy as dealing either with society as Confucianism or with nature or the cosmic Dào as Daoism. By contrast, traditional Chinese culture, like most other traditional ways of thinking and being in the world, simply does not recognize this division or hierarchy between humans and the rest of Heaven and Earth. Whether the enlightened person is managing or "putting in good order" (*zhì* 治) the individual body or the country, this always means aligning it with the larger environment by recognizing and resonating with the dominant forces of change in the macrocosm, which are in the present chapter conceptualized as Yīn and Yáng and the Five Dynamic Agents.

Sù Wèn Chapter 2, the "Great Discourse on Attuning the Body to the Four Qì" describes this capacity of the sages in similar terms:

Quotation from Sù Wèn[3]

唯聖人從之，故身無奇病，萬物不失，生氣不竭。

逆春氣，則少陽不生，肝氣內變。逆夏氣，則太陽不長，心氣內洞。
逆秋氣，則太陰不收，肺氣焦滿。逆冬氣，則少陰不藏，腎氣獨沈。

夫四時陰陽者，萬物之根本也。所以聖人春夏養陽，秋冬養陰。以從其根，故與萬物沈浮於生長之門。逆其根，則伐其本，壞其真矣。。。。

是故聖人不治已病，治未病，不治已亂，治未亂，此之謂也。

夫病已成而後藥之，亂已成而後治之，
譬猶渴而穿井，鬬而鑄錐，不亦晚乎。

Only sages accord with [the changes of the Dào]. Therefore, their bodies are not affected by unusual diseases, they do not lose harmony with the Myriad Things, and they do not exhaust their life-giving Qì.

If you go against the Qì of spring, Shàoyáng fails to [induce] sprouting and Liver Qì is affected by internal pathological changes. If you go against the Qì of summer, Tàiyáng fails to [induce] growth, and Heart Qì caves in internally. If you go against the Qì of autumn, Tàiyīn fails to [induce] harvest, and Lung Qì is scorched and full. If you go against the Qì of winter, Shàoyīn fails to [induce] storage, and Kidney Qì is turbid and sunken.

Now the Four Seasons and Yīn and Yáng are the root and foundation of the Myriad Things. For this reason, the sages nurture Yáng in the spring and summer and nurture Yīn in the autumn and winter. According with the root, you can rise and sink with the Myriad Things at the gate to sprouting and growth. Going against this root, you cut off the trunk and harm what is genuine!...

[3] *Sù Wèn* 《素問》 Chapter 2.

For this reason, the sages do not treat what is already diseased but treat what is not yet diseased, and do not put in order what is already in chaos, but put in order what is not yet in chaos. This is what I am talking about.

Now to have an illness that has already formed and only afterwards treat it with medication, to have chaos that has already formed and only afterwards put it in order, this is just like being thirsty and then digging a well, or to be in the middle of combat and then forging sharp weapons. Isn't it too late indeed at this point?

* * *

AGAIN WE CAN SEE HERE HOW ONCE AN ILLNESS MANIFESTS, MOST OF the battle is lost, and the wise person therefore directs their energy toward prevention, or in other words to aligning with the changes of the Dào in the macrocosm. In this context, what is the ultimate goal of medicine and medical intervention when practiced at its highest level? Clearly, the *Sù Wèn* is a text that reflects clinical experience and is intended as a guide for clinical application in the treatment of existing diseases as conditions of disorder (*luàn* 亂), where the physiological flow of Qì and Blood in the human body is disordered because the person is out of alignment with the cosmic Dào and therefore manifests certain signs and symptoms that need to be addressed. Nevertheless, it is important to always remember that the goal of Chinese medicine, whether expressed explicitly or not, in the early classics is to treat disease before it arises, or literally "to put in good order that which is not yet diseased" (*zhì wèi bìng* 治未病).

But if we do not want to limit ourselves to this negative expression of what the upper-level physician is not supposed to do, what is it that she or he should be aiming for instead? For an answer, we turn to the Preface to the *Shén Nóng Běncǎo Jīng* 《神農本草經》 (Divine Farmer's Classic of Materia Medica), another important Hàn dynasty classic.

Quotation from the Preface to the Shén Nóng Běncǎo Jīng 神農本草經序錄

上藥一百二十種為君，主養命以應天，無毒，
多服久服不傷人，欲輕身益氣不老延年者，本《上經》。

中藥一百二十種為臣，主養性以應人，無毒，
有毒，斟酌其宜，欲遏病補虛羸者，本《中經》。

下藥一百二十五種為佐使，主治病以應地，多毒，
不可久服，欲除寒熱邪氣、破積聚、愈疾者，本《下經》。

The upper-level medicinals consist of 120 types. These function as rulers. They are in charge of nurturing destiny and thereby resonate with Heaven. They are not poisonous and, [even] when taken in large quantities or over a long time, do not harm the person. If you want to lighten the body, boost Qì, avoid aging, and extend your lifespan, root [your prescriptions] in the upper [section of the] Classic.

The mid-level medicinals consist of 120 types. These function as vassals. They are in charge of nurturing the inner nature and thereby resonate with humanity. Some of them are poisonous and some are not, so deliberate their suitability carefully. If you want to check illness and supplement vacuity emaciation, root [your prescriptions] in the middle [section of the] Classic.

The lower-level medicinals consist of 125 types. These function as the assistants and messengers. They are in charge of treating illness and thereby resonate with Earth. In most cases, they are poisonous and may not be taken over a long period of time. If you want to eliminate the evil qì of cold and heat, break up accumulations and gatherings, and cure diseases, root [your prescriptions] in the lower [section of the Classic].

Even more clearly than the *Sù Wèn*, this citation from the Preface to the *Shén Nóng Běncǎo Jīng* spells out that treating disease (*zhì bìng* 治病) is the lowest form of medical practice, and that the appropriate role of the highest level of medicine is to "nurture destiny" (*yǎng mìng* 養命) in resonance with Heaven's activity, and of the mid level is to "nurture the inner nature" (*yǎng xìng* 養性) in resonance with human activity. A discussion of the full meaning of the terms *mìng* 命 and *xìng* 性 unfortunately transcends the limitations of this book. Here a short passage from *Zhuāngzi* might offer a partial answer while at the same time indicating the complexity that we are facing at this level of discourse:

Quotation from Zhuāngzi[4]

泰初有無，無有無名。一之所起，有一而未形。物得以生，謂之德。未形者有分，且然無間，謂之命。留動而生物，物成生理，謂之形。形體保神，各有儀則，謂之性。

In the very beginning, there is non-being, and there are no being and no names. In the place where the One arises, there is the One but not yet Form. What Things obtain and thereby are born, we call this Virtue-Power (dé). The state before Form has divisions and yet even so no spaces in between. This we call Destiny (mìng). Flowing movement then engenders Things, and Things, when completed, engender Guiding Principles. This we call Form (xíng). When the Form and the body foster the Shén, each having its models of conduct, this we call inner nature (xìng).

In a footnote to his translation of this passage, Fabrizio Pregadio explains: "Ming, literally translated above as 'mandate,' is the 'imprint' that Heaven confers to each entity, including its life span,

[4] *Zhuāngzi* 《莊子》 Chapter 12, *Tiān Dì* 天地 (Heaven and Earth).

its 'destiny' (also included in the notion of ming), its function in the world, and the assigned allotment of vital energy. Xing or 'nature' is the parcel of spirit (*shén*) that each living being harbors in its individuality, which the Zhuangzi here defines as 'form and body.'[5] Without diving too deeply into these difficult concepts, it suffices here to know that *mìng*, which literally means "order" or "decree" is in philosophical and medical literature associated with Heaven, whether we read it as "destiny," perhaps in the sense of a mandate from Heaven for our human existence in this lifetime, or in the more limited sense of "heavenly allotted lifespan." In contrast, *xìng* is our nature, as it is the nature of birds to fly and fish to swim, of gāncǎo to harmonize all other herbs and of fùzǐ to scatter cold and support yáng. In this context, it is the nature of humans to be social, love their family, and position themselves between Heaven and Earth.

In a simpler reading of the passage from the Preface to the *Shén Nóng Běncǎo Jīng*, we can translate *mìng* not as "destiny" (whatever that may mean), but as "lifespan," which is certainly one of the accepted meanings of this character in other contexts. We can then explain the highest category of medicinals to be involved in the pursuit of longevity and immortality, as an attempt to transcend the Earthly limitations of the human body by intentionally slowing down and even reversing the physiological process of aging that is a hallmark of ordinary human existence. These practices are generally referred to as "alchemy," whether in the external form as *wài dān* 外丹 or in the internal form as *nèi dān* 內丹. The second level of "nurturing the inner nature" in resonance with humanity can then be interpreted as the attempt to fulfill our social responsibilities, to nurture and express our unique abilities and characteristics in the service of humanity, in the sense of an activity that comes as naturally as a horse's gallop and a snake's slithering.

Now any contemporary practitioner of Chinese medicine has a choice to make: Do you want to humbly and sincerely embrace the lowest level of medical practice, that of treating disease in resonance

[5] Fabrizio Pregadio, *"Taoist Texts – Zhuangzi,"* www.goldenelixir.com/taoism/texts_zhuangzi.html, Nov. 28, 2017.

with the Earthly realm? Here it is important to recall that this is the scope of practice that the mainstream contemporary definition of medicine embraces and that its associated financial remunerations require. It is also the focus of what is being taught in our major clinical and academic professional institutions, what is tested in board exams, and what is expected by most patients on your treatment table. Any instance of diverging from this medical paradigm must be conscious and intentional, and be made clear to all participants, especially to the students and patients who are most likely expecting standard medical education and care.

Or do you want to dedicate your life to striving for the ideals outlined as the highest stage of medicine in the Classics, by tackling the steep ascent to the lofty realm of sagehood, let alone the transcendence of the perfected and accomplished persons? Are you prepared for the sacrifices, challenges, and loneliness that this lofty goal entails? Are you sure that you have what it takes to survive or even thrive in the challenging low-oxygen environment at those high elevations? And how do you reconcile that attempt at scaling the highest peak, which slowly but surely becomes more and more of a solitary pursuit, with the altruistic motivations that have brought most of us to Chinese medicine in the first place? As any serious mountain climber will warn you, you are sure to fail and perish if you attempt to climb Mount Everest without the many years of dedicated and single-minded training, abundant and sustained material, emotional, and spiritual support and guidance at home where you began your training, and then logistical assistance, companionship and support from people committed to your solitary success, and back-up plans in case of emergencies or unforeseen events at base camp. Statistically speaking, the majority of people are much better off enjoying the occasional picnic with a good cup of tea and a piece of cake on their local hillside or mountain range but otherwise live and work and play among their neighbors and family. For each of us, the answer to this question will differ, and it will most likely change in response to our experiences in this lifetime. We each need to decide individually how we can best be of service to Heaven, humanity, and Earth in our shared goal of living to the best of our ability to express our *xìng* nature and *mìng*

Destiny while at the same time being of assistance and value to our fellow human beings. There are no easy answers to this question, but that should not stop us from raising it honestly and earnestly, both within ourselves and with our colleagues, teachers, students, and perhaps even patients. As a terse book title by Paul U. Unschuld, one of the great contemporary translators of our profession, so aptly puts it, "What is Medicine?" is a question that needs to be addressed with care whenever we confront a medical paradigm so different from our own.[6]

[6] Paul U. Unschuld, *Was ist Medizin? Westliche und östliche Wege der Heilkunst* (Beck, 2003, published in English translation as *What is Medicine? Western and Eastern Approaches to Healing* (University of California, 2009).

Section Eighteen

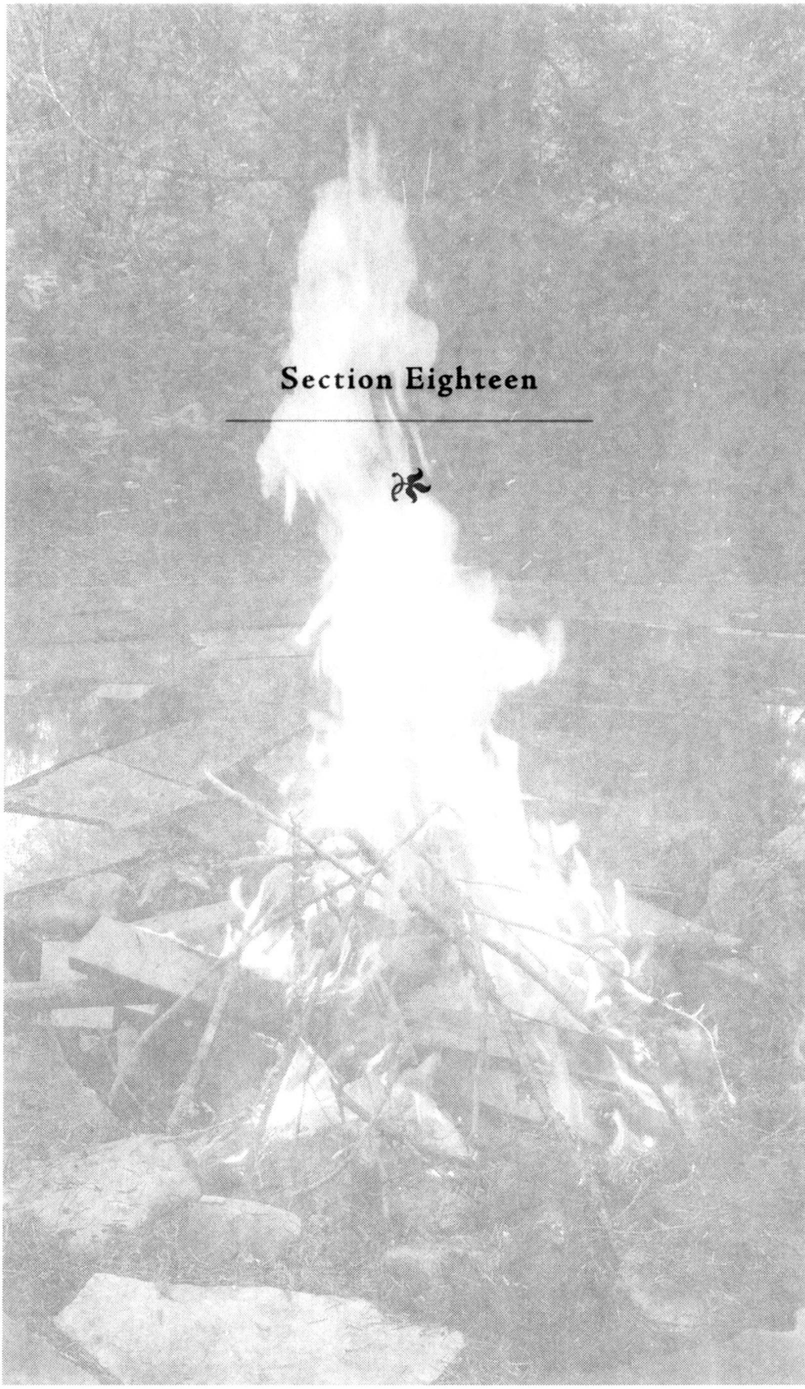

天氣通於肺，地氣通於嗌，風氣通於肝，雷氣通於心，
谷氣通於脾，雨氣通於腎。

Tiān qì tōng yú fèi,
dì qì tōng yú yì,
fēng qì tōng yú gān,
léi qì tōng yú xīn,
gǔ qì tōng yú pí,
yǔ qì tōng yú shèn.

The Qì of Heaven
communicates with the Lung,
the Qì of Earth
communicates with the throat,
the Qì of Wind
communicates with the Liver,
the Qì of thunder
communicates with the Heart,
the Qì of the valleys
communicates with the Spleen,
and the Qì of rain
communicates with the Kidney.

Commentary by Zhāng Zhìcōng 張志聰

『天氣通於肺』肺臟屬乎乾金，位居至高，而主周身之氣。故與天氣相通。此複言非惟頭之上竅通乎天。從腰以下以象地，而五臟六腑九竅六經，皆與天地之氣相通。惟賢人能法天之紀，用地之理以治身，故災害不能及也。

『地氣通於嗌』嗌乃胃腑之門。主受濕濁之氣以入胃。故與地氣相通。太陰陽明篇曰：喉主天氣、嗌主地氣。

『風氣通於肝』風生木，木生肝。外內之氣相通也。

『雷氣通於心』雷、火之發聲也。心為火臟，氣相感召，故與心相通。

『谷氣通於脾』脾為土臟，而主司轉運。谷氣、山谷之通氣也，故與脾氣相通。

『雨氣通於腎』腎為水臟。雨氣，寒水之氣也。

"The Qì of Heaven communicates with the Lung": The Lung Zàng Organ belongs to qián Metal and resides in the highest position, from where it rules the Qì all throughout the body. For this reason it communicates back and forth with the Qì of Heaven. This passage additionally states that it is not only the upper orifices in the head that communicate with Heaven. [The part of the body] from the lumbar region down resembles Earth, and the Five Zàng and Six Fǔ Organs and the Nine Orifices and Six Channels all communicate back and forth with the Qì of Heaven and Earth. Only paragons of virtue are able to conform to the threads of Heaven and apply the guiding principles of the Earth, to thereby manage their bodies. This is the reason why disasters and harm cannot touch them.

"The Qì of Earth communicates with the throat": The throat is the gate to the Stomach FǔOrgan. It is in charge of receiving the Qì of Dampness and Turbidity, which thereby enters the Stomach. For this reason, it communicates back and forth with the Qì

of Earth. As the chapter on the Tàiyīn and Yángmíng (Sù Wèn Chapter 29) *states, "The pharynx is in charge of Heaven's Qì; the larynx is in charge of Earth's Qì."*

"The Qì of Wind communicates with the Liver": Wind engenders Wood, and Wood engenders the Liver. This means that the Qì of the inside and the Qì of the outside communicate back and forth with each other.

"The Qì of thunder communicates with the Heart": Thunder is the sound produced by Fire. The Heart is the Zàng Organ of Fire, and because these two Qì resonate with and call out to each other, [thunder] communicates back and forth with the Heart.

"The Qì of the valleys communicates with the Spleen": The Spleen is the Zàng Organ of Earth and is in charge of overseeing conveyance. The Qì of the valleys is the joint Qì of the mountains and valleys; hence it communicates back and forth with Spleen Qì.

"The Qì of rain communicates with the Kidney": The Kidney is the Zàng Organ of Water. Rain Qì is the Qì of [winter-]Cold Water.

* * *

TO PRESENT THE STANDARD INTERPRETATION OF THIS PASSAGE and avoid merely repeating the ideas of my much wiser Chinese predecessors, I have translated Zhāng Zhìcōng's succinct yet insightful explanations below in full, line by line and phrase by phrase, for the associations between the human body and "Heaven and Earth" offered in this Section. Beyond that, the only parts of this passage that require additional comments are these three terms:

The explanation by Zhāng below shows that the character *yì* 嗌 can have two meanings: In its standard, more general sense, it is used to refer to the throat as a whole and is equated in Chinese dictionaries with *yān hòu* 咽喉, the upper and lower parts of the throat respectively, which is then, in contemporary Chinese medical literature and English dictionaries of biomedicine and TCM, further explained in anatomical terms as the pharynx and larynx. In addition, in the pronunciation of *aì*, the character 嗌 carries the meaning of choking from a food blockage in the throat, which is significant in the present context. The equation by Chinese commentators of *yì* 嗌 with *yán hòu* 咽喉 makes sense as long as we translate it as "throat" and understand these other two terms as referring to the upper and lower part of the throat, rather than blindly accepting their contemporary English anatomical terms. The key contrast between *yì* 嗌 and *hòu* 喉 that we need to grasp to appreciate Zhāng's explanation below for the association of *yì* with the Stomach is that this opposition is not related to their location, as the upper and lower part of the throat, but to their physiological function: As such, *yì* refers to the part of the throat that is associated with the transport of food and drink, or in other words, the pharynx and the upper part of the esophagus, while *hòu* is the part of the throat associated with breathing, or in Chinese medicine terms, with the transport of Qì, which means the pharynx and larynx. Viewed from this angle, the association of *hòu* with Heaven Qì and *yì* with Earth Qì, and hence with the Stomach, begins to make sense. Wáng Bīng's commentary on this line even suggests translating *yì* as esophagus in its entirety instead of as throat, or the esophageal part of the throat: "The lung resides in a high position, and thus Heaven Qì connects with it. The *yì* is next in the body below it, and thus Earth Qì connects with it (肺居高，故天氣通;嗌次下，故地氣通。)."

In addition, the expression *gǔ qì* 谷氣, which I have translated above as "Qì of the valleys," similar to both Paul U. Unschuld and Hermann Tessenow, and Elisabeth Rochat de la Vallée's versions, requires a note: Zhāng Zhìcōng makes it clear, in his commentary cited below, that he also reads the character as "valley" by using the compound *shān gǔ* 山谷 "mountains and valleys." It is, however, also possible, as many contemporary Chinese commentators and scholar-physicians do, to read 谷 as a short form for 穀 "grain," which was already a common substitution in medical and other literature from the classical period and also happens to be the modern simplified version of the traditional character. Associating the Spleen with grain is certainly an easy and clinically tempting connection to make. Nevertheless, we can also follow Wáng Bīng in emphasizing that "Valleys are empty. The spleen receives and takes in and therefore communicates with valleys" (谷空虛，脾受納，故通谷). Furthermore, valleys are the low places in the mountains, and the Spleen is the *Zàng* Organ associated with lowliness and with emptiness that receives the Essence of Water and Grain in the same way that valleys receive the water running off the mountains. As such, both readings have their merits.

Lastly, I have added the word "[winter-]" before "Cold water" in Zhāng's commentary on the association between rain and the Kidney to add a bit of clarity for Western readers. The reason for my choice is that the term used here for cold, *hán* 寒, has the specific meaning of cold in the winter season, as evidenced by the inclusion of *bīng* 冫 "ice" in the character. My addition is also meant to tease out the connection of the kidney not just with fluids or "water" in general but also with darkness, depth, blackness, winter-cold, and the most intimate and hidden spaces and processes, like a mountain cave with no exit, a bottomless abyss, or the deepest part of a lake. The kidney, and with it the reproductive organs and processes, are the human body's manifestation of the fuzzy consciousness of a hibernating bear in the middle of winter; of the fertile period of hidden storage in winter before the outburst of creativity in the spring; and of the layer of fertile black humus in the deeper layers of the soil where plants deposit their seeds, grow their roots, and prepare to launch their bright green shoots from when the warm spring winds start blowing.

While the explanations provided in this commentary are very helpful, it is interesting to contemplate where this information came from, especially considering the neat lists of Five-Phase and Six-Channel associations that we find elsewhere. The grouping here of Heaven, Earth, Wind, Thunder, Valleys, and Rain does not fit into any of the standard correlations that I am aware of and includes a pair of unusual contrasts (Heaven and Earth and Lung and Throat, respectively); three climatic factors of which only Wind fits into the standard medical lists in its correlation with the Liver; and then the mysterious "Qì of Valleys" associated with the Spleen. In addition, we can logically explain the association of rain with the Kidney as being about its physiological function of managing the fluids, but in standard medical literature the climatic factor closest to rain is Dampness (*shī* 濕), which is never associated with the Kidney but with Spleen-Earth. We do find the Five *Zàng* Organs all represented here, but in addition we have the odd association of the Qì of Earth with the throat. Even after Zhāng's explanation that the throat stands here for the Stomach as the sole *Fǔ* Organ, we are still left puzzling over the reasons for including what is usually a minor part of the body that is mentioned only in passing.

六經為川，腸胃為海，九竅為水注之氣。

Liù jīng wéi chuān,
cháng wèi wéi hǎi,
jiǔ qiào wéi shuǐ zhù zhī qì.

The Six Channels constitute rivers, the Intestines and Stomach constitute seas, and the nine orifices constitute [the places] where Qì pours out like water.

Commentary by Zhāng Zhìcōng 張志聰

『六經為川』六經、手足三陰三陽之經脈也。外內環轉如川流之不息。

『腸胃為海』腸胃受盛水穀，如海之無所不容。又胃為水穀之海而外合海水；腸為受盛之官。

『九竅為水注之氣』精氣通上竅。濁水出下竅。

"The Six Channels constitute rivers": The Six Channels are the three Yīn and three Yáng vessels of the hands and feet. Outside and inside, they circulate [fluids] like the ceaseless flow of rivers.

"The Intestines and Stomach constitute seas": The Intestines and Stomach receive Water and Grain in abundance, like the sea's limitless ability to contain [all water flowing into it]. Additionally, the Stomach is the Sea of Water and Grain and matches the ocean water on the outside, while the Intestines constitute the Office of Receiving Plenitude.

"The Nine Orifices constitute [the places] where Qì pours out like water": Essence Qì penetrates up to the upper orifices, while turbid Water exits through the lower orifices.

For readers unable to read the Chinese source text out loud, it is also important to realize that all the phrases in this line conform to exactly the same grammatical and rhythmic pattern of five characters and are thus clearly meant to be read as a unit:

。。。氣通於。。。

… Qì communicates with …

This sentence pattern changes abruptly in the next line to one of four characters, with the exception of the longer third phrase, where two-character body features are identified with geographical terms:

○○○為○○○

...constitute...

A brief side note may be in order here to explain a visual play with words in the Chinese source text that can be lost on modern readers who are not familiar with ancient or sloppy handwritten versions of the characters: The character *chuān* 川 ("rivers") is actually a part of the character *jīng* 經 ("channels"), as is more obvious in its alternate form 巛. In the early versions of both of these characters, the element appears as three parallel wavy lines, depicting flowing water.

Lastly, readers unfamiliar with classical terminology may need a reminder that the Nine Orifices are generally defined as the seven orifices in the head (two ears, two eyes, two nostrils, and the mouth), which are in charge of discharging clear Yáng, and the anterior and posterior Yīn orifices below (urethra and anus), which are in charge of eliminating turbid Yīn. This is most likely also the definition intended by the original authors of *Sù Wèn* Chapter 5. An alternative explanation of the term *jiǔ qiào* 九竅, however, is presented in the discussion of the Qì of the Five *Zàng* Organs in the *Nàn Jīng*:

Quotation from Nàn Jīng 難經[1]

五臟者，當上關於九竅也。故肺氣通於鼻，鼻和則知香臭矣；肝氣通於目，目和則知黑白矣；脾氣通於口，口和則知穀味矣；心氣通於舌，舌和則知五味矣；腎氣通於耳，耳和則知五音矣。

The Five Zàng Organs should above be gated by the Nine Orifices. As such, Lung Qì connects to the nose, and when the nose is harmonious, we know good and bad smells. Liver Qì connects to the eyes, and when the eyes are harmonious, we know black and white. Spleen Qì connects to the mouth, and when the mouth is harmonious, we know the flavor of Grains. Heart Qì connects to the tongue, and when the tongue is harmonious, we know the Five Flavors. Kidney Qì connects to the ears, and when the ears are harmonious, we know the Five Sounds.

Regardless of whether one counts the mouth and tongue as a single orifice, or counts the nose as two nostrils, the numbers do not add up above. Whatever we make of this small incongruence, it is generally accepted that the Nine Orifices in the present context include the Yīn orifices in the lower body. In addition, Zhāng Jièbīn argues that the order of characters should be reversed from 水注之氣 "where Qì pours out like water" to 水氣之注 "where water and Qì pour out."

[1] *Nàn Jīng* 《難經》 (Classic of Difficulties) Chapter 37.

以天地為之陰陽，陽之汗，以天地之雨名之；
陽之氣，以天地之疾風名之。

Yǐ tiān dì wéi zhī yīn yáng,
yáng zhī hàn,
yǐ tiān dì zhī yǔ míng zhī;
yáng zhī qì,
yǐ tiān dì zhī jí fēng míng zhī.

Taking Heaven and Earth to
serve as [models for] Yīn and Yáng,
Yáng sweat is named after the rain
of Heaven and Earth,
and Yáng Qì is named
after the quick-moving Winds
of Heaven and Earth.

* * *

Commentary by Zhāng Zhìcōng 張志聰

『以天地為之陰陽』陰陽者，天地之道也。以天地之道通乎身之陰陽。

『陽之汗，以天地之雨名之。』汗出於陰液，由陽氣之宣發，故曰陽加於陰謂之汗。雨乃地之陰濕，亦由天氣之所化施，故可方人之汗。

『陽之氣，以天地之疾風名之。』風出於地之隧谷，陽氣發於裡陰。以疾風名之者，言陽氣之行身有道，無少逆滯者也。

"Taking Heaven and Earth to serve as [models for] Yīn and Yáng...": Yīn and Yáng are the Dào of Heaven and Earth. Through this Dào of Heaven and Earth, they connect with the Yīn and Yáng of the body.

"...Yáng sweat is named after the rain of Heaven and Earth": Sweat comes from the Yīn fluids [but] relies on the diffusing and effusing action of Yáng Qì. As such I say that when Yáng is added onto Yīn, we refer to this as sweat. Now rain is the Yīn Dampness of the Earth, but also relies on being transformed and distributed by Heaven's Qì. Hence we can liken it to sweat in humans.

"...Yáng Qì is named after the quick-moving Winds of Heaven and Earth": Wind comes out of the tunnels and ravines of the Earth, [and similarly] Yáng Qì effuses from the interior Yīn. The fact that it is named after the quick-moving wind is saying that the action of Yáng Qì in the body has pathways and does not have a shortage of countercurrent flow and obstructions.

* * *

暴氣象雷，逆氣象陽。
故治不法天之紀，不用地之理，則災害至矣。

Bào qì xiàng léi,
nì qì xiàng yáng.

Gù zhì bù fǎ tiān zhī jì,
bù yòng dì zhī lǐ,
zé zāi hài zhì yǐ.

Fulminant Qì is a manifestation of thunder; Countercurrent Qì is a manifestation of Yáng.

Therefore, if treatment does not conform to the structural arrangements of Heaven and does not apply the organizing patterns of Earth, calamity and disaster are sure to arrive!

* * *

Commentary by Zhāng Zhìcōng 張志聰

『暴氣象雷，逆氣象陽』：氣暴如雷火之發，氣逆如陽熱之勝。此複言陽氣之如風行於上下四旁，無暴無逆也。

***"Fulminant** Qì is a manifestation of thunder; countercurrent Qì is a manifestation of **Yáng"**: Qì [can be] fulminant like the eruption of thunder and Fire, and it can move **countercurrent**, like a prevalence of Yáng Heat [which causes pathological upward **movement**]. This is again saying that the movement of Yáng Qì up and down and in **all** four directions like the wind [should] not be fulminant or countercurrent.*

* * *

The first part of Section Eighteen describes normal and healthy processes both in the natural environment and in the human body. Beginning with the mentioning of "quick-moving winds" in the second half of Section Eighteen, however, the text turns toward what are generally considered harmful processes, whether as natural phenomena (quick-moving winds) or at the level of the body as fulminant or countercurrent Qì. The position of sweat here right in the middle, and its association with the clearly beneficial but potentially disastrous natural phenomenon of rain, reminds us of the dual nature of sweat. Like rain, it is the result of a complex finely tuned interaction between Yīn Qì emerging from the depth and Yáng Qì acting at the surface in processes of evaporation, condensation, and precipitation. As any farmer can (but probably won't because it is so obvious) tell you, rain at regular and predictable intervals, in response to certain seasonal factors, is essential to a thriving balanced ecosystem, but excessive unseasonal rain can quickly cause life-threatening flooding and erosion and earth movements that destroy fields, carry off soil and plants, and drown plant life. Similarly, sweating is an important mechanism for thermal balancing and releasing excess heat, pathological factors, or waste products through the surface of the body, the absence of which must be addressed with strong treatments to promote sweating, but it can also easily deplete Essence and fluids or have dire consequences when it is inhibited. As we will see in the next section, this turn towards pathology introduces the final part of the *Great Discourse*, which discusses pathological factors and their treatment.

When we read the present Section Eighteen as a whole, the description of concrete resonances between the macrocosmic body of Heaven and Earth and the human microcosmic body reminds me of a statement ascribed to Sūn Sīmiǎo 孫思邈 in his biography, which is in turn reminiscent of a similar earlier passage in the *Bàopǔzǐ* 抱朴子:

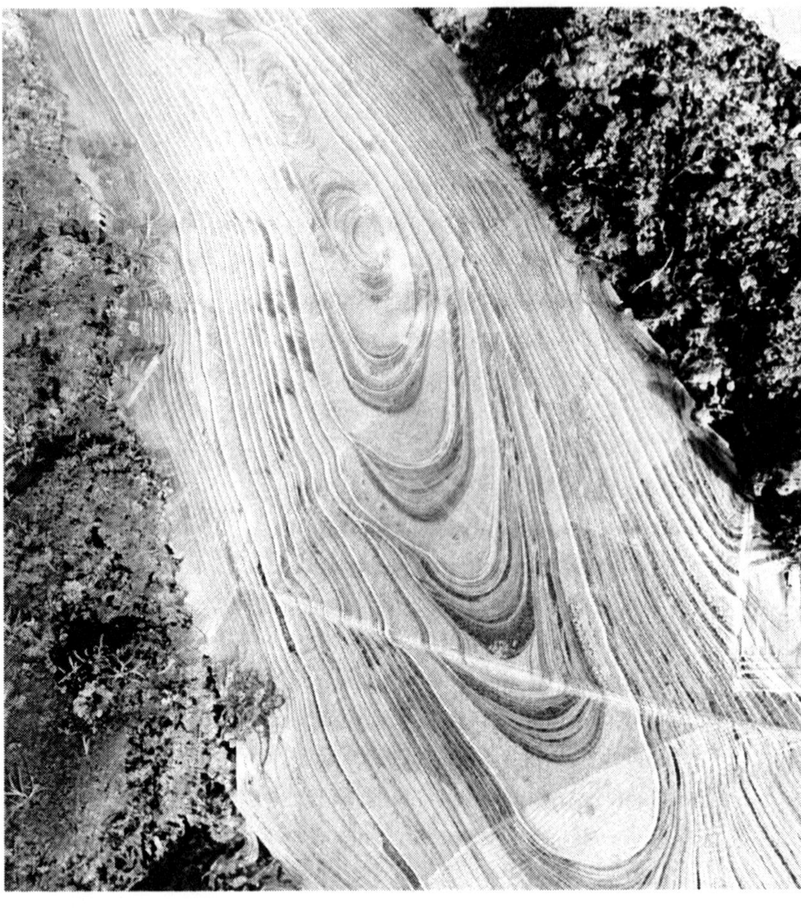

Quotation from the Jiù Táng Shū[2]

照鄰有惡疾，醫所不能愈，乃問思邈：名醫愈疾，其道何如？
思邈曰：吾聞善言天者，必質之於人；善言人者，亦本之於天。
天有四時五行，寒暑迭代，其轉運也，和而為雨，怒而為風，
凝而為霜雪，張而為虹蜺，此天地之常數也。

人有四肢五臟，一覺一寐，呼吸吐納，精氣往來，流而為榮衛，
彰而為氣色，發而為音聲，此人之常數也。

陽用其形，陰用其精，天人之所同也。及其失也，蒸則生熱，否則生寒，結而為瘤贅，陷而為癰疽，奔而為喘乏，竭而為焦枯。診發乎面，變動乎形。

推此以及天地亦如之。故五緯盈縮，星辰錯行，日月薄蝕，孛彗飛流，此天地之危診也。寒暑不時，天地之蒸否也。石立土踴，天地之瘤贅也。山崩土陷，天地之癰疽也。奔風暴雨，天地之喘乏也。川瀆竭涸，天地之焦枯也。

良醫導之以藥石，救之以針劑。聖人和之以至德，
輔之以人事。故形體有可愈之疾，天地有可消之災。

Zhào-Lín had a malignant illness which physicians were unable to cure, so he went and asked Sīmiǎo: "What principles do the famous physicians employ to cure illness?" Sīmiǎo answered: "I have heard that if one is skilled at talking about Heaven, one must substantiate it in the human realm; if one is skilled at talking about humans, one must also root it in Heaven. In Heaven, there are Four Seasons and Five Dynamic Agents; winter-cold and summerheat alternate with each other. When this cyclical revolution is harmonious, it forms rain; when it is angry, wind; when it congeals, frost and snow; when it stretches out, rainbows. These are the constancies of Heaven and Earth.

[2] *Jiù Táng Shū* 《舊唐書：孫思邈傳》 (Old Táng Documents: Biography of Sūn Sīmiǎo).

Humans have Four Limbs and Five Zàng Organs. They alternate between being awake and sleeping. In exhaling and inhaling, spitting out and sucking in, Essence and Qì come and go. In their flow, they constitute Yíng provision and Wèi defense, they manifest as complexion, and they erupt as sound. These are the constancies of humanity.

Yáng employs the Form, Yīn employs the Essence. This is where Heaven and humanity are identical. When [the constancies] are lost, if [Qì and Essence] steam upward, they cause Heat; if they are blocked, they cause Cold; if they are bound, tumors and excrescences; if they sink, abscesses; if they scatter wildly, panting and dyspnea; and if they are exhausted, scorching and withering. Their symptoms arise on the face, and their transformations move around in the body.

When one extends this analogy to apply it to Heaven and Earth, it is also likewise. Thus the waxing and waning of the Five Planets, the irregular motions of the constellations, the eclipses of the sun and moon, the flight of shooting stars, these are Heaven and Earth's symptoms of danger. Unseasonable winter-cold and summer-heat are the ascent or blockage [of Qì and Essence] in Heaven and Earth. Uprighted boulders and thrust-up earth are the tumors and excrescences of Heaven and Earth. Collapsing mountains and caved-in ground are the abscesses of Heaven and Earth. Scattered winds and violent rains are the panting and dyspnea of Heaven and Earth. Dried-up streams and parched marshes are the scorching and withering of Heaven and Earth.

An excellent physician guides [Qì] with medicines and [lancing] stones and rescues with needles and prescriptions. A sage[ly ruler] harmonizes [Qì] to perfect his power and uses this as support in order to manage the affairs of humanity. Thus, the human body has illnesses that can be cured, and Heaven and Earth have calamities that can be dispersed."

* * *

From this perspective of the Heaven-Humanity-Earth (*tiān rén dì* 天人地) triad, and picking up from our discussion of the previous section, what is the proper role of the physician, what is the ultimate goal of any medical treatment, and what are the most appropriate skills and tools that any healer should hone both in terms of diagnosis and treatment? And related to the nature of the text we are attempting to decipher and translate into contemporary clinical application here, what are the purpose and intended audience of a text like the present *Great Discourse on the Resonant Manifestations of Yīn and Yáng*?

Speaking just from personal experience, I used to read especially the early chapters of the *Sù Wèn* more as a cosmological and philosophical text, or as a beautiful work of literature in its own right, than as clinically relevant information. This is unfortunately also the position advocated by the majority of contemporary practitioners of Chinese medicine in the West. I also used to argue that the authors of the *Nèi Jīng* as a whole must have consulted professional physicians and other healers or incorporated their texts but were more likely to be a part of the Hàn emperor's inner circle of literati bureaucrats who were interested in the human body primarily to gain insights from the management of one microcosm to apply to the management of another microcosm, namely the state. After teaching this material for many years to students of Chinese medicine and discussing it with my clinical colleagues, however, I am more and more convinced that a deep understanding of the equivalence between microcosm and macrocosm, and of the natural laws that govern the changes in both of them, is vital to a practice of Chinese medicine that unleashes its full potential while staying true to its roots. As the text warns, "if treatment does not conform to the structural arrangements of Heaven and does not apply the organizing patterns of Earth, calamity and disaster are sure to arrive!"

Section Nineteen

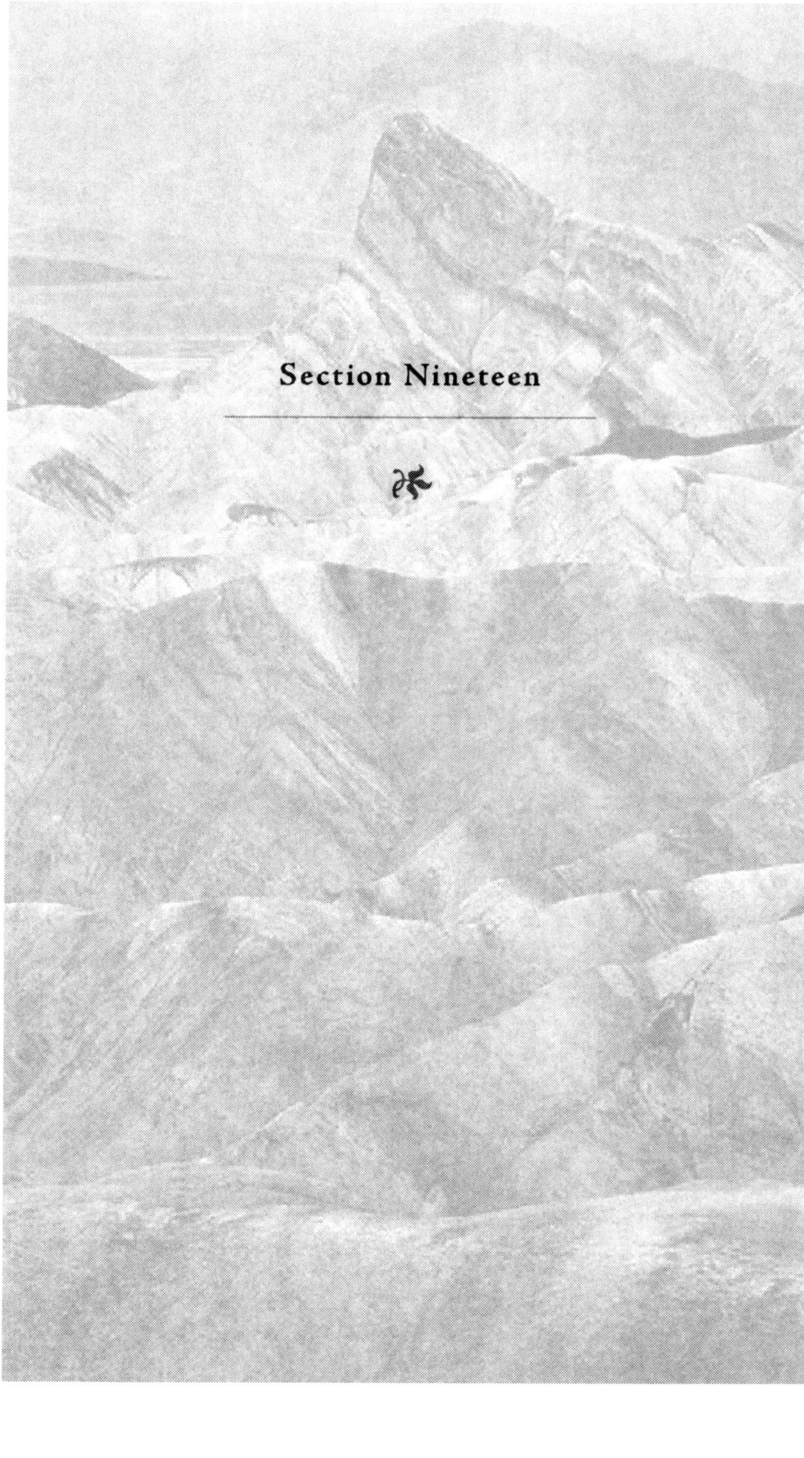

故邪風之至，疾如風雨。故善治者治皮毛，其次治肌膚，其次治筋脈，其次治六腑，其次治五臟。治五臟者，半死半生也。

Gù xié fēng zhī zhì, jí rú fēng yǔ.
Gù shàn zhì zhě zhì pí máo,
qí cì zhì jī fū, qí cì zhì jīn mài,
qí cì zhì liù fǔ, qí cì zhì wǔ zàng.

Zhì wǔ zàng zhě,
bàn sǐ bàn shēng yě.

As such, the arrival of Evil Wind
is quick-moving like wind and rain.
As such, skillful practitioners treat
the skin and body hair;
less skillful practitioners treat the flesh;
practitioners even less skillful treat
the Sinews and Vessels;
ones less skillful yet treat the
Six Fǔ Organs; and ones less skillful
yet treat the Five Zàng Organs.

Practitioners who treat
[disease at the level of] the
Five Zàng Organs will have
half their patients die
and half survive.

THE REPEATED USE OF *FĒNG* 風 IN THE FIRST SENTENCE MAY befuddle the reader at first but can easily be explained as referring in the first instance to its occurrence in the human body, or in other words to Wind as a pathology in the technical medical sense, which I have therefore emphasized by means of capitalization, and to wind as a natural phenomenon in the second instance.

Commentary by Wáng Bīng 王冰

至謂至於身形。治皮毛，止於萌也。治肌膚，救其已生。治筋脈，攻其已病。治六腑，治其已甚。治五臟，治其已成。神農曰：病勢已成，可謂半愈。然初成者獲愈，固久者伐形。故治五臟者，半死半生也。

To arrive means to arrive at the person's body. To treat the skin and body hair means that you stop the disease when it is just germinating. To treat the flesh means that you rescue what has already sprouted. To treat the Sinews and Vessels means that you attack what has already become a disease. To treat the Six Fǔ Organs means that you treat what has already become serious. To treat the Five Zàng Organs means that you treat what has already matured. The Divine Farmer said, "When the disease dynamic has already matured, we can call this 'recovery of half.'" This being so, in the initial stages of maturity you can still achieve recovery, but once it has become consolidated and chronic, it will knock down the Form. Therefore, treating disease in the Five Zàng Organs results in half the patients dying and half surviving.

* * *

AT FIRST SIGHT, THE SENTIMENT ABOVE THAT THE HIGHEST-LEVEL practitioners treat the most superficial level of the body while the least skillful ones treat the deepest level at the Five *Zàng* Organs contradicts everything Chinese medicine students learn in their first introductory class. They are, after all, constantly reminded to "treat disease at the root" or "treat disease by pursuing it in the trunk/foundations" (治病比求於本), as the very introduction to this whole chapter puts it. Addressing disease at the level of the skin seems to be the exact opposite of "treating the root," or pursuing disease to the deepest level. How do we explain this? There are two ways we can address this conundrum, both of which can contribute helpful insights to medical practice:

First, we can explain this statement here by placing it in the correct historical context. In classical China, physicians were judged by the outcome of their treatments. With no licensing body or institutional supervision, a physician's reputation was his most important asset. As such, it was of utmost importance that physicians honed their diagnostic skills so that they could get away as far as they could from patients whose the disease had penetrated so far into the body that they would be unable to cure them. The story of Biǎn Qùe 扁鵲 attempting to treat Duke Huán 桓 of Qí 齊 when the latter's disease was still at the level of the texture lines in the skin (*còu lǐ* 腠理) has already been cited above (see page 65.) As you may remember, the famous physician's warnings were ignored by the Duke who therefore refused treatment and instead accused Biǎn Què of profiteering. As a result, the disease progressed to penetrate more and more deeply into his body, until Biǎn Qùe decided to abruptly flee the state, explaining his departure with this final statement: "When the disease was residing in the texture lines of the flesh and skin, it could have been reached with hot liquids and hot compresses. When the disease was residing in the blood vessels, it could have been reached with needles and stones. When it was in the intestines and stomach, it could have been reached with medicinal liquors and wines. But once it is in the bones and marrow, not even the Divine Commander of Destiny can do anything about it. Now that your disease is in the bones and marrow, your servant therefore has no reason to pay you his respects." In a place and time where physicians were blamed directly for the outcome of their treatments, it makes perfect sense that an important key to success was the ability to assess the severity of a patient's condition and predict the outcome of treatment by the ability to determine how deeply the disease had progressed into the body, so that one could refuse to treat patients who were determined to be too risky. From this perspective, it makes sense that the skilled practitioner treats disease where it is the easiest to address and most certain to respond positively to treatment, namely at the most superficial level of the skin and body hair, and at the same time avoids patients with an unpredictable treatment outcome where the disease has already progressed to the deeper levels, in the same way that Biǎn Què refused to help Duke Huán in the final stage of his disease.

The progression of disease from the skin and body hair to the flesh to the sinews and vessels to the Six *Fǔ* Organs to the Five *Zàng* Organs is similar but slightly different to other accounts of disease progression, such as the one found in the "Discourse on the Essentials of Needling" (*Sù Wèn* Chapter 50). There, each of the levels is associated with one of the Five *Zàng* Organs, progressing from the Lung (skin) to the Spleen (flesh), to the Heart (Vessels), to the Liver (Sinews) to the Kidney (bones), and then to the marrow, which lacks a Five-*Zàng* correlation.

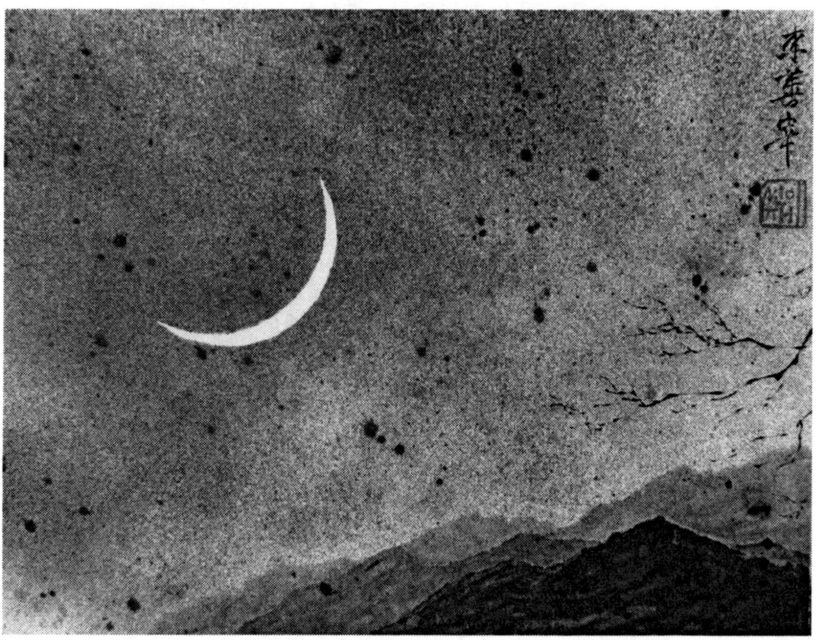

※ ※ ※

Quotation from Sù Wèn[1]

淺深不得，反為大賊，內動五臟，後生大病。

故曰：病有在毫毛腠理者，有在皮膚者，有在肌肉者，
有在脈者，有在筋者，有在骨者，有在髓者。

是故刺毫毛腠理無傷皮，皮傷則內動肺，肺動則秋病溫瘧，泝泝然寒栗。

刺皮無傷肉，肉傷則內動脾，脾動則七十二日四季之月，病腹脹煩不嗜食。

刺肉無傷脈，脈傷則內動心，心動則夏病心痛。

刺脈無傷筋，筋傷則內動肝，肝動則春病熱而筋弛。

刺筋無傷骨，骨傷則內動腎，腎動則冬病脹腰痛。

刺骨無傷髓，髓傷則銷鑠胻痠，體解㑊然不去矣。

[1] *Sù Wèn* 《素問》 Chapter 50, *Discourse on the Essentials of Needling* 《刺要論》.

If you do not achieve the [appropriate] depth [in needling], [your treatment] will instead be a great robbery, internally stir the Five Zàng Organs, and afterwards generate serious illness.

Therefore I say that among diseases, there are those that are located in the fine body hair and texture lines of the còulǐ, those that are located in the skin, those that are located in the flesh, those that are located in the vessels, those that are located in the sinews, those that are located in the bones, and those that are located in the marrow.

For this reason, when needling the fine body hair and còulǐ, avoid injuring the skin. Injury to the skin internally stirs up the lung, and a stirred-up lung causes the patient to fall ill with warm malaria with shivering and cold shudders in the fall.

When needling the skin, avoid injuring the flesh. Injury to the flesh internally stirs up the spleen, and a stirred-up spleen causes the patient to fall ill with abdominal distention, vexation, and lack of appetite during the 72 days of the intercalary months.

When needling the flesh, avoid injuring the vessels. Injury to the vessels internally stirs up the heart, and a stirred-up heart causes the patient to fall ill with heart pain in the summer.

When needling the vessels, avoid injuring the sinews. Injury to the sinews internally stirs up the liver, and a stirred-up liver causes the patient to fall ill with heat [effusion] and slackness of the sinews in the spring.

When needling the sinews, avoid injuring the bones. Injury to the bones internally stirs up the kidney, and a stirred-up kidney causes the patient to fall ill with distention and lumbar pain in the winter.

When needling the bones, avoid injuring the marrow. Injury to the marrow results in the frailness of a chronic illness, soreness in the calves, and sluggishness and fatigue, which you cannot get rid off."

* * *

故天之邪氣，感則害人五臟；水穀之寒熱，感則害于六腑；地之濕氣，感則害皮肉筋脈。

Gù tiān zhī xié qì, gǎn zé hài rén wǔ zàng; shuǐ gǔ zhī hán rè, gǎn zé hài yú liù fǔ; dì zhī shī qì, gǎn zé hài pí ròu jīn mài.

As such, contracting the evil Qì of Heaven results in injury to the person's Five Zàng Organs; contracting Cold and Heat of Water and Grain results in injury to the Six Fǔ Organs; and contracting Dampness Qì of Earth results in injury to the skin, flesh, Sinews, and Vessels.

The relationship between disease causes and their penetration into the human body is obviously a highly significant one in light of the previously stated notion that skilled physicians avoid treating disease that has penetrated more deeply into the body. This is particularly pressing in cases when disease must be treated in the Five *Zàng* Organs, a level where only half the patients are said to survive. In practical terms, however, how do we reconcile these two notions and yet see any hope for the function of the physician and the efficacy of medical treatment? The answer to this question hinges partly on how we define "the evil Qì of Heaven." In accordance with standard terminology, this simply refers to climatic factors that make us ill, or in other words weather patterns that do not follow the normal patterns of change in the sky. This is already spelled out by Wáng Bīng:

* * *

Commentary by Wáng Bīng 王冰

其四時之氣，八正之風，皆天邪也。《金匱真言論》曰：八風發邪以為經風，觸五臟，邪氣發病。故天之邪氣，感則害人五臟。熱傷胃及膀胱，寒傷腸及膽氣，故感則害於六腑。濕氣勝則榮衛之氣不行，故感則害於皮肉筋脈。

In this context, the Qì of the Four Seasons and the Winds of the Eight Directions are all evils from Heaven. Sù Wèn Chapter 4 (The Discourse on the Perfected Words from the Golden Cabinet) states: "The Eight Winds erupt as evil, thereby becoming Wind in the Channels and accosting the Five Zàng Organs, and [thus] evil Qì erupts as disease. As such, Heaven's Qì, when contracted, harms the person's Five Zàng Organs. Heat injures the Stomach and Bladder, while Cold injures the Intestines and Gallbladder Qì. As such, they harm the Six Fǔ Organs when contracted. When Dampness Qì prevails, the Qì of yíng Provisioning and wèi Defense fails to move. As such, [dampness Qì] harms the skin, flesh, Sinews, and Vessels, when contracted.

* * *

Gāo Shìzōng reiterates this sentiment and equates this "evil Qì of Heaven" with the standard list of what are usually referred to as the Six Excesses (*liù yín* 六淫) of Wind, Cold, Summerheat, Dampness, Dryness, and Fire. These are called the "creators of the hundred diseases" (*bǎi bìng zhī shēng* 百病之生) in *Sù Wèn* Chapter 74.

* * *

Commentary by Gāo Shìzōng 高士宗

上文皮肌筋脈腑臟之病，有因於天者，有因於地者，有因於人者，故天之邪氣，感於人身，則害人五臟。邪氣，風寒暑濕燥火也。人之水穀之寒熱，感於人身，則害六腑。水穀寒熱，飲食失宜，或寒或熱也。 地之濕氣，感於人身，則害皮肉筋脈，因於濕者，下先受之，故曰地之濕氣。

In the text above, among disease conditions in the skin, flesh, Sinews, Vessels, Fǔ Organs, and Zàng Organs, there are those that are caused by Heaven, those that are caused by Earth, and those that are caused by Humanity. As such, when the evil Qì of Heaven affects the person, it harms the Five Zàng Organs. Evil Qì here means Wind, Cold, Summerheat, Dampness, Dryness, and Fire. When Cold or Heat from the Water and Grain of Humanity affect the human body, they harm the Six Fǔ Organs. Cold or Heat from Water and Grain means that food and drink have lost their suitability, whether [because they are too] cold or too hot. When Dampness Qì of the Earth affects the body, it harms the skin and flesh and tendons and Vessels. When disease is due to Dampness, it is first received in the lower body, and therefore we say it is Dampness Qì of Earth.

* * *

What does this statement mean in concrete terms and in clinical practice? The associations of Dampness with the superficial level of the body, and of food and drink with the Six *Fǔ* Organs, as entering more deeply, are easy to follow. And theoretically speaking, we can explain this statement from the perspective of the resonances between the macrocosm, as the triad of Heaven, Humanity, and Earth, and the microcosm of the human body, divided into the three layers of *Zàng* Organs, *Fǔ* Organs, and the superficial structures of the body, going from the inside out. Nevertheless, it is a basic, and presumably unavoidable, human experience to be affected negatively by the influences of the climate, as we experience in each "flu season." Are we to conclude that the ancient Chinese were simply so much more attuned to their external environment that they managed to avoid invasions of these pathogenic environmental factors much more frequently than our weakened modern bodies protected by air conditioning and central heating? Or are we, along with countless generations of Chinese commentators, misunderstanding the meaning of "evil Qì of Heaven" here? Since neither of these explanations are satisfying to me, it is perhaps best to read this line here as separate from and unrelated to the previous section, best to read this line here as separate from and related to the previous section, especially since that section discussed treatment while we are focusing on etiology. This is my reason for breaking up Section Nineteen in the way that I have done here. With the following lines, we return to the discussion of treatment principles in the physician's effort to "attune Yīn and Yáng."

Section Twenty

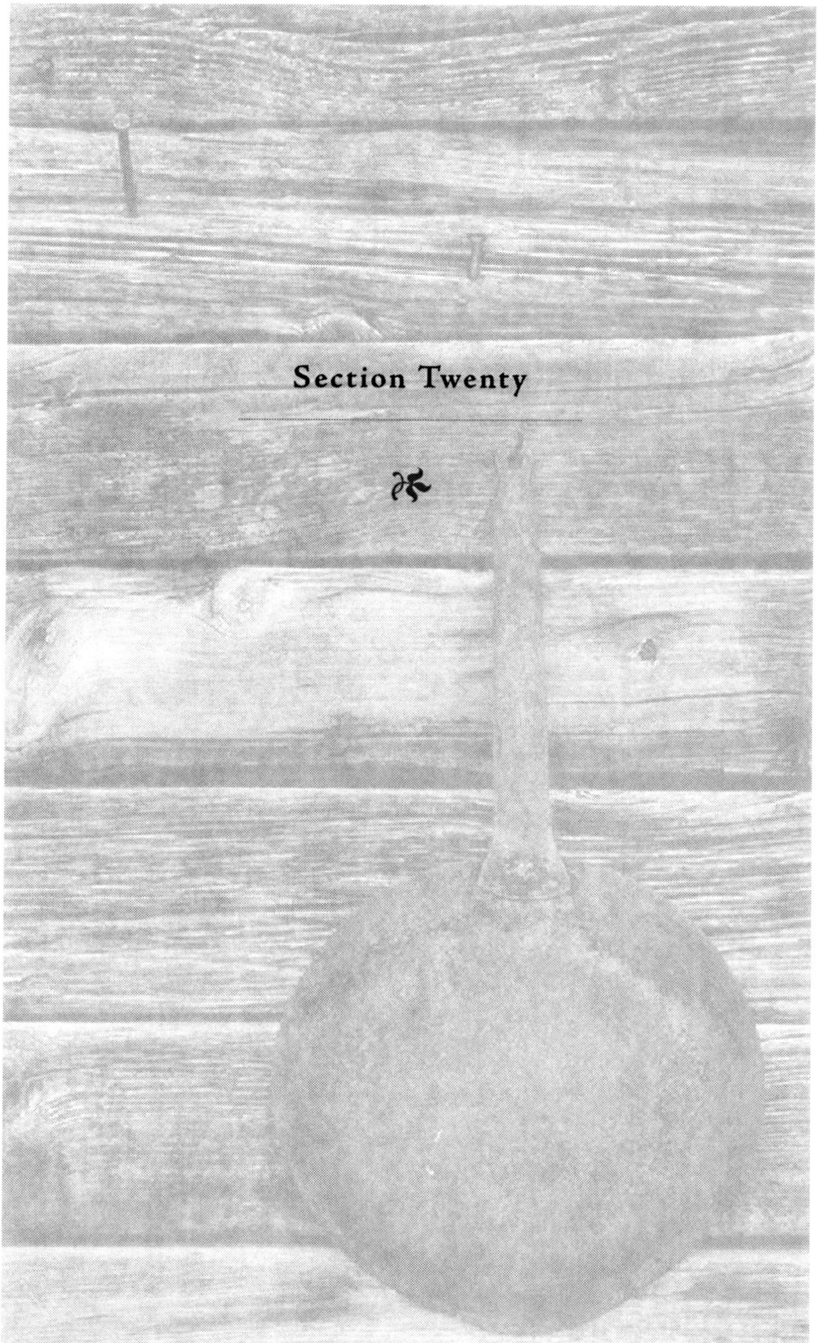

故善用針者，從陰引陽，從陽引陰，以右治左，
以左治右，以我知彼，以表知裡，以觀過與不及之理，
見微得過，用之不殆。

Gù shàn yòng zhēn zhě,
cóng yīn yǐn yáng, cóng yáng yǐn yīn,
yǐ yòu zhì zuǒ, yǐ zuǒ zhì yòu,
yǐ wǒ zhī bǐ, yǐ biǎo zhī lǐ,
yǐ guān guò yǔ bù jí zhī lǐ,
jiàn wēi dé guò, yòng zhī bù dài.

As such, practitioners who
are skilled at using needles
[observe the following guidelines:] from
the Yīn guide the Yáng,
from the Yáng guide the Yīn;
by the right treat the left,
by the left treat the right;
from their own [experience]
know the other; and from
the exterior know the interior.
By [thus] contemplating the underlying
pattern of excesses and insufficiencies
[in the patient's body], they see the
subtle [signs] and obtain
[control over] what is in excess.
Their use [of needles]
does not carry any risk!

THIS PASSAGE MENTIONS A NUMBER OF TREATMENT METHODS that deserve additional explanation and can and have been interpreted in different ways by different commentators and translators. I have therefore attempted to keep my translation above as literal as possible to allow readers to make up their own mind. My notes below simply present some possibilities, based on standard readings. Of course we can also follow Wáng Bīng's laconic comment on the first line that "all of these are deeply illuminated methods for using needles" (凡此皆深明用鍼之法也) and leave it at that. Mǎ Shì's commentary, however, should be a little more helpful. While lengthy, it manages to express the underlying sentiment that ties all these phrases together with both elegance and clinical insight.

Commentary by Mǎ Shì 馬蒔

上文言由皮毛而漸入臟腑，則在外為表，在內為裡，在表為陽，在裡為陰。善用鍼者，知陽病必行于陰也，故從陰以引之而出於陽，知陰病必行于陽也，故從陽以引之而入于陰。

《難經》六十七難曰：五臟募皆在陰，而俞在陽者何謂也？然。陰病行陽，陽病行陰，故令募在陰，俞在陽。此乃指背腹為陰陽，特一端耳，然鍼法之從陰引陽，從陽引陰，不止於此。

《靈樞》終始、禁服、四時氣篇人迎脈盛為陽經病，則瀉陽補陰;氣口脈盛為陰經病，則瀉陰補陽。補瀉施而陰陽和，亦從陰引陽，從陽引陰法也。

凡人身經絡，左與右同，我與彼同，表與裡同，故以右治左，以左治右，以我知彼，以表知裡，如繆刺論以邪之入於經者為巨刺，流溢於大絡而生奇病者為繆刺。繆刺者，以左取右，以右取左。其所謂大絡者，十五絡也；巨刺者，正刺也；繆刺者，與經脈異處也。

Since the text above starts from the skin and body hair and gradually enters into the Zàng and Fǔ Organs, this means that the location on the outside constitutes the exterior, and the location on the inside the interior, and that the location in the exterior constitutes Yáng and the location in the interior constitutes Yīn. The person who is skilled at using needles knows that Yáng disease must move into the Yīn, and as such draws it from the Yīn to exit in Yáng; and knows that Yīn disease must move into the Yáng, and as such draws it from the Yáng to enter the Yīn.

The 67th Difficulty in the Nàn Jīng states: "All the Mù Alarm Points of the Five Zàng Organs are located in Yīn, and all the Shū Transport Points are located in Yáng. What do we mean by this?" Answer: "Yīn disease moves into Yáng, and Yáng disease moves into Yīn. For this reason, the Mù Alarm Points are in Yīn, and the Shū Transport Points are in Yáng." This passage points only to this particular perspective, that the back and the abdomen are Yīn and Yáng. Nevertheless, the needling method of "guiding the Yáng from the Yīn and guiding the Yīn from the Yáng" is not limited to this [meaning] alone.

In the Líng Shū 靈樞 Chapters 9, 19, and 42, an abundant pulse at Rényíng means disease in a Yáng channel, in which case you drain Yáng and supplement Yīn; an abundant pulse at Qìkǒu means disease in a Yīn channel, and then you drain the Yīn and supplement the Yáng. The application of supplementing and draining and the harmonization of Yīn and Yáng, these are the method of "drawing the Yáng from the Yīn and drawing the Yīn from the Yáng."

Always in the channels and network vessels of the human body, the left and right are identical, the person's own [experience] and the other's are identical, and the exterior and the interior are identical. As such we treat the left by means of the right and treat the right by means of the left; know the other by means of our own [experience]; and know the interior by means of the exterior. This is just like in the "Discourse on Baffling Needling" (Sù Wèn Chapter 63) where if the evil has entered the Channels, it means Grand Needling, but if it has poured into the large Network Vessels and engendered strange diseases, it means Baffling Needling. Baffling Needling means to choose the right for the left and to choose the left for the right. What this text refers to as the "large network vessels," are the fifteen Network Vessels. Grand Needling means straight needling, while Baffling Needling means that the location is different from the flow in the channels.

* * *

If the reader is not familiar with the method of "baffling needling" (*miù cì* 繆刺), *Sù Wèn* Chapter 63 is an entire chapter devoted to this topic. Grand Needling (*jù cì* 巨刺) is one of the Nine Needling Methods (*jiǔ cì* 九刺) described in *Líng Shū* 靈樞 Chapter 7 as needling evil in the Channels by treating the right from the left and the left from the right side of the body. To differentiate between the indications for Grand Needling, which refers to deeper needling of Channels, and Baffling Needling, which is a more superficial needling technique of the Network Vessels, I quote the introduction from the "Discourse on Baffling Needling," *Sù Wèn* Chapter 63:

* * *

Quotation from Sù Wèn[1]

黃帝問曰：余聞繆刺，未得其意，何謂繆刺？

岐伯對曰：夫邪之客於形也，必先舍於皮毛，留而不去，入舍於孫脈，留而不去，入舍於絡脈，留而不去，入舍於經脈，內連五臟，散於腸胃，陰陽俱感，五臟乃傷，此邪之從皮毛而入，極於五臟之次也，如此則治其經焉。今邪客於皮毛，入舍於孫絡，留而不去，閉塞不通，不得入於經，流溢於大絡，而生奇病也。夫邪客大絡者，左注右，右注左，上下左右與經相干，而布於四末，其氣無常處，不入於經俞，命曰繆刺。

帝曰：願聞繆刺，以左取右以右取左奈何？其與巨刺何以別之？

岐伯曰：邪客於經，左盛則右病，右盛則左病，亦有移易者，左痛未已而右脈先病，如此者必巨刺之，必中其經，非絡脈也。 故絡病者，其痛與經脈繆處，故命曰繆刺。

The Yellow Emperor asked: "I would like to hear about Baffling Needling. I have not yet grasped its significance. What do you mean by Baffling Needling?"

[1] *Sù Wèn* 《素問》 Chapter 63, *miù cì lùn* 繆刺論 (The Discourse on Baffling Needling)

Qí Bó replied: "The way evil intrudes through the Form is first by lodging in the skin and body hair. If it remains instead of leaving [the body], it enters more deeply to lodge in the Grandchild Vessels. If it remains instead of leaving, it enters more deeply to lodge in the Network Vessels. If it remains instead of leaving, it enters more deeply to lodge in the Channels, which are internally linked to the Five Zàng Organs. Dispersing in the Intestines and Stomach, Yīn and Yáng are both affected, and the Five Zàng Organs are injured. This is this order in which evil enters from the skin and body hair and finally ends up in the Five Zàng Organs. If it is like this, then you treat the affected Channels. In the present case, evil has intruded through the skin and body hair and entered more deeply to lodge in the Grandchild Vessels. Remaining [in the body] instead of leaving, it has become blocked and congested without moving freely, and is unable to enter the channels, pouring into the Great Network Vessels and engendering strange diseases there. Now when evil intrudes into the Great Network Vessels, it pours from the left to the right, and from the right to the left, up and down and left and right interfering with each other in the Channels and spreading to the four tips. Its Qì has no constant location and does not enter the Channel Transport Shū Points. This is [the situation] that Baffling Needling refers to."

The Emperor said: "I would like to hear about Baffling Needling. Why is it that you choose the right [side of the body] for treating [evil] in the left and the left [side of the body] for treating [evil] in the right? And how do you distinguish it from Grand Needling?"

Qí Bó replied: "As evil intrudes into the Channels, exuberance in the left results in disease in the right, and exuberance in the right results in disease in the left. Moreover, there are also conditions that shift and move around, or cases where pain on the left has not yet stopped but the pulse on the right first [indicates] disease. Situations like these are ones where you must [treat the disease by] Grand Needling, and you must strike the Channels, and not the Network Vessels. As such, in diseases of the Network Vessels, the pain and the channel pulses are in baffling locations and therefore this method is called Baffling Needling."

* * *

Whether we read Yīn and Yáng here as referring to the inner and outer layers of the body, the front and the back, the upper and lower body or the Yīn and Yáng pairs of Channels, or even as repletion and vacuity and draining and supplementing, the key point of this section is that Yīn and Yáng must always be in a state of dynamic equilibrium. An exuberance or defect in one aspect will have an opposite but equally detrimental effect on its counterpart, with the involvement of an external evil or without. The skilled acupuncturist knows how to recognize the precise nature of the disturbance and is thereby able to choose the perfect countermeasure by knowing which needling technique to employ without damaging the surrounding structures. As always, the key is to scrutinize with subtlety so that disorder can be recognized and addressed before it has had a chance to sprout and penetrate more deeply into the body or escalate with a cascade of resulting symptoms. In this way, one's treatment will not carry any risk!

* * *

Commentary by Z'ev Rosenberg on "Contrary Needling"

In Denver, Colorado, where I had a busy clinic in the 1980's, I used to see a lot of skiing accident cases. One case stands out in my mind, a young man in his mid twenties who I had treated for other issues, who broke his right leg skiing and had his leg set in a cast from his foot to his groin. As the leg was healing, he had a lot of bone-, tendonal, muscular pain. Since I could not treat the affected leg, I remembered reading about contrary needling in an early textbook,[2] translated by Dan Bensky, sourced from a reference in *Sù Wèn* Chapter 5. This was long before I had a reliable translation of the *Sù Wèn* available (just Henry Lu's was available in those days). So following this lead, I needled the opposite leg (left) at GB 34, 41, and Spleen 6, then completed the pattern on the right arm with TB 5 and LI 4. There was

[2] *Acupuncture: A Comprehensive Text (*Shanghai College of Traditional Medicine).

immediate relief of the leg pain! We continued treatments, which as it turns out contributed to healing faster than the Western doctors had expected. I used the same strategy in treating broken arms with further success.

* * *

善診者，察色按脈，先別陰陽；審清濁，而知部分；視喘息，聽音聲，而知所苦；觀權衡規矩，而知病所主；按尺寸，觀浮沉滑澀，而知病所生以治。

無過以診，則不失矣。

Shàn zhěn zhě, chá sè àn mài, xiān bié yīn yáng; shěn qīng zhuó, ér zhī bù fèn; shì chuǎn xī, tīng yīn shēng, ér zhī suǒ kǔ; guān quán héng guī jǔ, ér zhī bìng suǒ zhǔ; àn chǐ cùn, guān fú chén huá sè, ér zhī bìng suǒ shēng yǐ zhì.

Wúguò yǐ zhěn, zé bù shī yǐ.

Practitioners who are skilled at diagnosis investigate the complexion and palpate the flow in the vessels, to first differentiate Yīn and Yáng; scrutinize the clear and the turbid, to thereby know the specific location and level [of the disease]; observe the breathing and listen to the sounds [produced by the patient], to thereby know the location of suffering; contemplate the weights and balance beam [of scales] and the compass and the square, to know what governs the disease; and palpate the chǐ and the cùn pulse and contemplate its floating or sunken, slippery or rough quality, to thereby know what has produced the disease, and thereby [they are able to] treat it.

Because they make no mistakes in their diagnosis, they do not miss anything!

Moving on to the next passage, the text emphasizes the importance of careful diagnosis so that any imbalance or dysfunction in the body can be addressed as early and with as minimal intervention as possible. In other words, it is an elaboration on the basic premise of classical Chinese medicine that the skilled physician "treats disease before it arises" 治未病. In this context, it emphasizes the subtle skills of facial diagnosis and pulse reading in particular. By knowing from experience what a healthy pulse should feel like in each season, for example, the skillful practitioner can detect a potential imbalance when that special quality is lacking or overshadowed by a different quality at that time.

Commentators disagree on the exact meaning of the second phrase, "scrutinize the clear and the turbid, to thereby know the specific location and level" (審清濁，而知部分). According to most commentators, the "clear and turbid" refers to the color of the patient's skin. By distinguishing whether it is bright, light, and clear, or dark, deep, and murky, the skillful practitioner can determine whether the disease is located in the Yáng or Yīn aspect of the body, respectively. It is up to debate whether Yīn and Yáng here refer to the *Zàng* and *Fǔ* Organs, or to Yīn and Yáng aspects of the Vessels, or to the Blood and Qì, or are meant simply as general terms to a deeper, more serious, and a more superficial and easily treated condition.

Further on, we encounter another difficult phrase, "contemplate the weights and balance beam [of scales] and the compass and the square" (權衡規矩). These are two common pairs of nouns, both referring to instruments of measuring and here used because of their function of creating balance and perfect alignment. A more elegant and less literal translation of this line might then start "By contemplating balance and perfect alignment, they know…" Nevertheless, as another possible interpretation, many commentators read these four nouns as referring to the four seasonal qualities of the pulse, in other words, to the specific characteristics of the pulse that should indicate that the patient's body is in alignment with the seasonal changes in the macrocosm. This reading is suggested by the following passage in Sù Wèn Chapter 17.

Quotation from Sù Wèn[3]

以春應中規，夏應中矩，秋應中衡，冬應中權 。

In spring, [the pulse] should accord with the compass, in the summer with the L-square, in the fall with the balance beam of a scale, and in the winter, with the weights of a scale.

In other words, the proper pulse should be rounded like a compass in the spring, like a carpenter's square in the summer, level like the balance beam on a perfectly weighted scale in the fall, and heavy and deep like the weights of a scale, or like a stone sinking into a pond in the winter.

Contemplating these four qualities or characteristics is said to allow the practitioner to "know what governs the disease." The character *zhǔ* 主, which I have translated as "governs," is commonly used in medical literature in the sense of "indication." So you could translate it here as "...they know [the specific treatments] indicated for the disease." Alternatively, you could also read this line as "they know what [evil] is ruling over the disease." My translation above is purposely worded in such a way as to leave both possibilities open. Considering the likely reference to the seasonal pulse qualities in previous phrase, it might refer to the seasonal Qì that is ruling the disease.

[3] *Sù Wèn* 《素問》 Chapter 17, *Mài Yào Jīng Wēi Lùn* 脈要精微論 (Discourse on the Essential Subtleties of the Pulse).

Section Twenty-One

故曰：病之始起也，可刺而已；其盛，可待衰而已。
故因其輕而揚之，因其重而減之，因其衰而彰之。
形不足者，溫之以氣；精不足者，補之以味。

Gù yuē: Bìng zhī shǐ qǐ yě,
kě cì ér yǐ; qí shèng, kě dài shuāi ér yǐ.

Gù yīn qí qīng ér yáng zhī,
yīn qí zhòng ér jiǎn zhī, yīn qí
shuāi ér zhāng zhī.

Xíng bù zú zhě, wēn zhī yǐ qì;
jīng bù zú zhě, bǔ zhī yǐ wèi.

Therefore it is said:
'When a disease is just beginning
to arise, it can be needled and stopped.
When it is flourishing, you can merely
wait for it to weaken, and then stop it.'

Thus, relying on the lightness
[of a condition], lift it up to scatter it;
relying on the heaviness
[of a condition], curtail it [gradually];
relying on the weakness
[of a condition], make it apparent.

When the Form is insufficient,
warm it by means of Qì.
When the Essence is insufficient,
supplement it by means of Flavor.

THE FIRST LINE OF THIS LAST SECTION OF THE *GREAT Discourse* is yet another restatement of the rule to "treat disease before it arises" (*zhì wèi bìng* 治未病), here expressed in terms of treatment efficacy. The fact that disease is easy to treat and responds quickly when in its very incipient stage but much more difficult or perhaps even impossible to address later on, when it has developed into a full-blown condition, is one of the fundamental premises of public health. It can be applied to everything from prenatal care to pollution control to removing diet sodas from school lunches. It is obviously related to the second line at the very beginning of the *Great Treatise*, that "To treat disease, you must seek it in the basics," which in the context of this *Discourse* refers to understanding and restoring the balance between Yīn and Yáng. In this way, the end of the *Great Discourse*, while much more clinically-oriented than the lofty beginnings, take us right back to where we started.

Commentary by Mǎ Shì 馬蒔

此言善治者之有序也。方知病之始起也，其邪未盛，可即刺之，而病自已。其邪盛者，可待其勢之既衰以刺之，而病亦已。

夫病之始起而刺之即已，所謂因其病勢之輕而發揚之耳。如下文其在皮者汗而發之，及其盛而必待其衰，所謂因其病勢之重而漸減之也。至於末後，則病勢既衰，當因其邪氣之衰，而使正氣之彰。斯則初中末三治之法，所謂初則發攻，中則調和，末則收補者是也。

治病者可不知哉？然本節雖言用鍼，而用藥之理亦不外是也。

This section speaks to the fact that people who are skilled at treatment have a sequence [in their treatment methods]. When they become aware of the very beginning of an illness, when the disease evil is not yet exuberant, they can instantly needle it, and the disease is spontaneously finished. When the evil is exuberant, they can only wait for its force to weaken before they can needle it, and then the disease is also finished.

Now the situation where a disease at its very beginning is needled and immediately stopped, this is what is meant by the rule to rely on the lightness of the disease force to lift it up to scatter it. Likewise in the text below, the advice to effuse a disease by sweating when it is located in the skin and to have to wait for it to weaken when it has become exuberant, this is what is meant by the rule to rely on the seriousness of the disease force to gradually curtail it. Arriving at the tail end afterwards then, the disease force is now weakened, and we should now rely on the weakness of its evil Qì and then cause Right Qì to become apparent. These are the three treatment methods for the beginning, middle, and end [stages of a disease], which is what we mean by effusing and attacking in the beginning, attuning and harmonizing in the middle, and gathering in and supplementing in the end.

How could anybody treating disease not know this? This being so, even though the present chapter speaks of using needles, the guiding principles of using medicinals do not fall outside of this either.

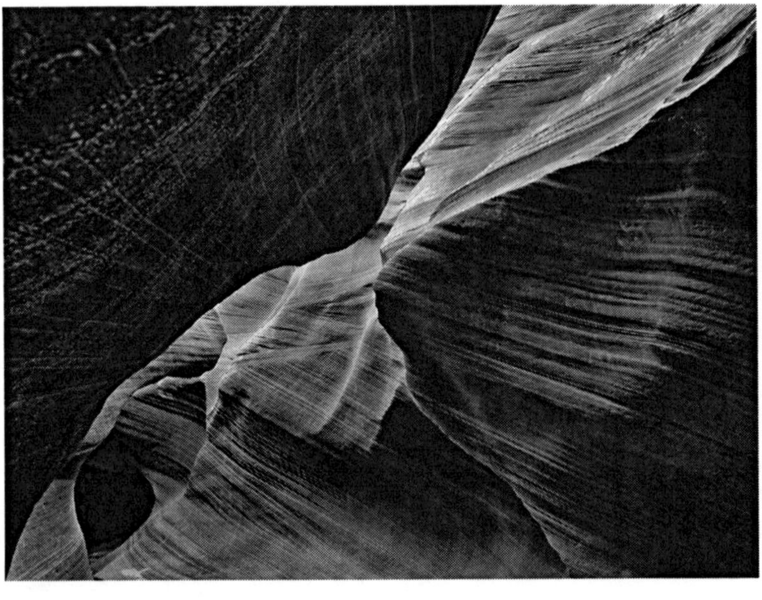

As Mǎ Shì here emphasizes, the treatment principle outlined in the beginning of this Section can be applied not only to acupuncture but to any other treatment modality as well. Regarding my translation above, the reader should be made aware that the two-character phrase *ér yǐ* 而已, which I have translated above as "and stop" or "and be stopped," can be read in two different ways. As a compound at the end of a statement, it has the meaning of "and that is all," or "and that is all there is to it." But read as two separate characters, as I have done above to translate it consistently in both occurrences in the first line, it can also be translated as "and then it is finished/stopped." Specifically, *yǐ* 已 can be a verb meaning "to stop," or "to finish," which can here be read in the active sense as "and then [the doctor] stops it" or passive as "and then [the disease] is stopped." In the use of the phrase *ér yǐ* in the first line, however, it is important to recognize this implied meaning of "that's all there is to it," in the sense that you simply needle the disease in the very beginning and thereby stop it, with no need to do or worry about anything else, while in the second phrase there is nothing else you can do but wait for the disease to weaken on its own, before you can apply treatment through needling to stop it.

In the next passage, the character *yáng* 揚 means literally "to raise something up to make it fly" (飛舉也), according to the *Shuō Wén Jiě Zì* dictionary. One of its more common meanings is thus, for example, to winnow grain. Here, I read the character as meaning to dissipate a disease that is characterized by "lightness," whether we interpret that quality as meaning that it is still superficial, not critical yet, or more literally as "light" in the sense of being close to the surface and easy to lift. In either case, it is easily treated by lifting it up and scattering it. An example of this kind of treatment would be Gégēn Táng 葛根湯 on the first or second day of Cold Damage conditions.

In the second phrase of that line, "relying on the heaviness [of a condition], curtail it [gradually]," the character *jiǎn* 減 (curtail), should be replaced with 瀉, "to drain," according to Zhāng Jièbīn and others. Other commentators have interpreted the character as referring to a gradual approach of diminishing the condition bit by bit when it has reached a state of being "critical," which is another possible reading of *zhòng* 重, besides literal heaviness, or characterizing a repletion-type

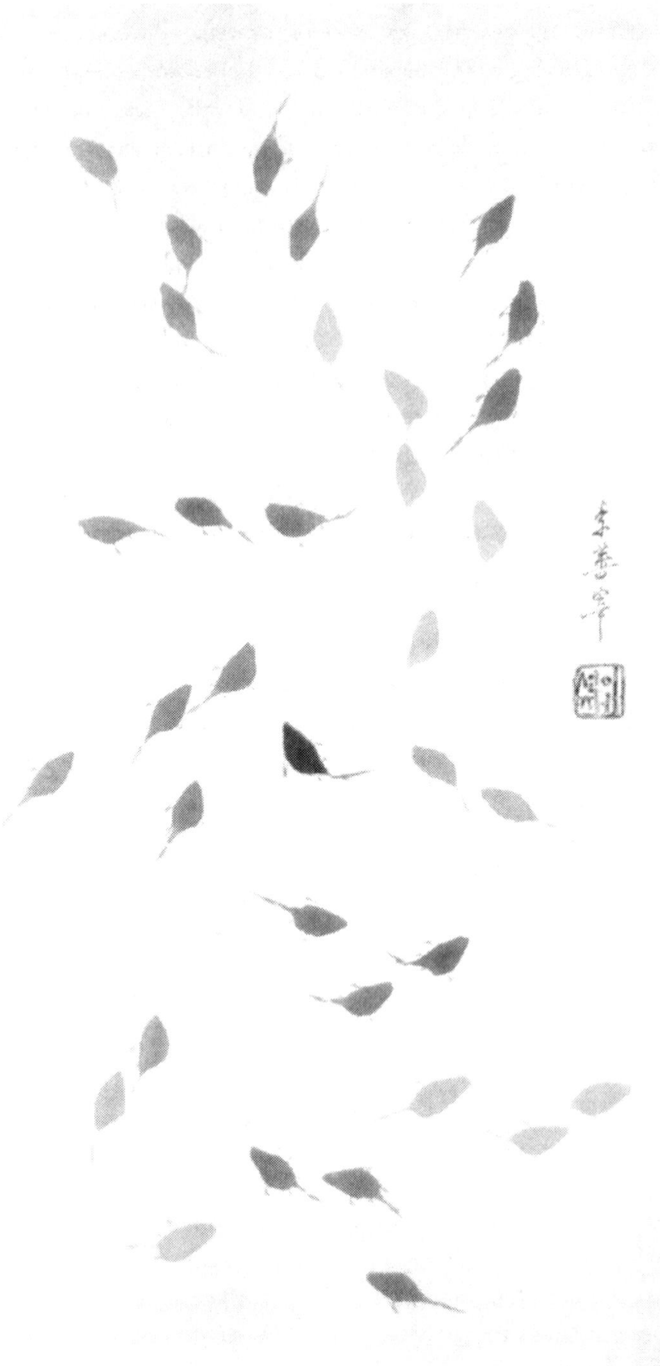

disorder that is located deeper in the interior. Lastly, it has been pointed out that this entire middle phrase may be a mistake since *yáng* 揚 and *zhāng* 彰 rhyme, while *jiǎn* 減 does not fit this pattern. Moreover, the surrounding lines contain pairs of opposites instead of patterns of triplets. The character *jiǎn* 減 literally means "to reduce," "to diminish," as in the *Shuō Wén Jiě Zì* definition as "to decrease" (損也). It is sometimes used interchangeably with its close relative *jiǎn* 减, which refers more specifically to subtracting something or lessening the severity or degree, a meaning that fits the present context perfectly.

In the last phrase of the second line, I have translated the character *zhāng* 彰 as "to make apparent," in the literal sense of "to manifest something." Depending on whether the direct object "it" is taken to refer to the disease evil or to the weakened Qì and Blood of the patient, commentators have explained its meaning quite differently. Elisabeth Rochat de la Vallée translates it as "restore resplendence," while Paul U. Unschuld and Hermann Tessenow has "let it shine again." Zhāng Jièbīn explains weakness here as referring to "vacuity of Qì and Blood" (*qì xuè xū* 氣血虛), which should be treated by making it resplendent again through supplementing and boosting treatments.

其高者，因而越之；其下者，引而竭之；中滿者，瀉之於內。
其有邪者，漬形以為汗；其在皮者，汗而發之；其慓悍者，按而收之；其實者，散而瀉之。

Qí gāo zhě, yīn ér yuè zhī;
qí xià zhě, yǐn ér jié zhī;
zhōng mǎn zhě, xiè zhī yú nèi.

Qí yǒu xié zhě, zì xíng yǐ wéi hàn;
qí zài pí zhě, hàn ér fā zhī;
qí piāo hàn zhě, àn ér shōu zhī;
qí shí zhě, sàn ér xiè zhī.

If it is located in an elevated position, dissipate it. If it is located below, draw it [down] and exhaust it. If it is a case of fullness in the center, drain it internally.

If there is a presence of evil involved, soak the Form in order to make the patient sweat. If [the disease] is located in the skin, effuse it by sweating. If [the disease] is quickly moving and ferocious, constrain it by applying pressure. If [the disease] is [marked by] repletion, drain it by scattering it.

The standard interpretation of the advice to dissipate disease when elevated, to draw it down and exhaust it when located below, and to drain it internally in cases of fullness in the center is that it recommends inducing vomiting for conditions located in the upper body, inducing purgation through diarrhea for conditions in the lower body, and getting rid of center fullness by internally dispersing it. "Center" has been explained either as referring to the Middle *Jiāo*, i.e., to the location between above and below, or to something deep on the inside, as opposed to the exterior level of the body. Given the context here, I incline towards the first of these interpretations.

審其陰陽，以別柔剛。陽病治陰，陰病治陽，定其血氣，
各守其鄉，血實宜決之，氣虛宜掣引之。

Shěn qí yīn yáng, yǐ bié róu gāng.
Yáng bìng zhì yīn, yīn bìng zhì yáng,
dìng qí xuè qì, gè shǒu qí xiāng,
xuè shí yí jué zhī, qì xū yí chè yǐn zhī.

Scrutinize Yīn and Yáng in order to
differentiate softness and hardness.
In Yáng disease, treat the Yīn;
in Yīn disease, treat the Yáng.
Settle the patient's Blood and Qì
so that each is safeguarded
in its own territory.
When the Blood is replete,
it is appropriate to dredge it;
when the Qì is vacuous,
it is appropriate to tug and pull it.

* * *

Commentary by Gāo Shìzōng 高士宗

凡此施治之法，當審其陰陽，以別柔剛。陰陽者，
天地之道也，柔剛者，乾剛坤柔，亦天地之道也。

陽盛則陰虛，故陽病當治其陰，陰盛則陽虛，故陰病當治其陽。

定其血氣，定其病之在血在氣也。各守其鄉，血病勿使傷氣，氣病勿
使傷血也。血實宜決之，勿使傷氣矣，氣虛宜掣引之，勿使傷血矣。

此一節，言人身之陰陽形體，而應象於天地，
是當法天地之陰陽，以為延醫之善也。

Always in these methods of applied treatments, we must scrutinize the patient's Yīn and Yáng in order to differentiate softness and hardness. Yīn and Yáng: They are the Dào of Heaven and Earth. Softness and Hardness: Qián (☰ ䷀ the name of the trigram and hexagram associated with Heaven) being hard and Kūn (☷ ䷁the name of the trigram and hexagram associated with Earth) being soft, they are also the Dào of Heaven and Earth. Yáng exuberance results in Yīn vacuity, and therefore we must treat the patient's Yīn in cases of Yáng disease. Yīn exuberance results in Yáng vacuity, and therefore we must treat the patient's Yáng in cases of Yīn disease.

Settling the patient's Blood and Qì means settling whether the disease is located in the Blood or in the Qì. Each being safeguarded in its own territory means that in Blood disease, do not allow it to injure the Qì, and in Qì disease, do not allow it to injure th Blood. In Blood repletion, it is suitable to dredge it, but you must not allow it to injure Qì. In Qì vacuity, it is suitable to tug and pull it, but you must not allow it to injure the Blood!

This section explains how Yīn and Yáng in the human body resonate with the manifestations in Heaven and Earth and how they must conform to Yīn and Yáng in Heaven and Earth. Through these [resonances] we extend the skill of medicine!

* * *

Commentary by Z'ev Rosenberg

The importance of understanding the nuances and oscillations of Yīn and Yáng is repeated over and over again in *Sù Wèn* Chapter 5. What is clear is that the physician needs to understand this blueprint of Yīn and Yáng, and its manifestations first in Heaven and Earth, and then solidified in the human organism. One of the treatment methods mentioned in the *Shāng Hán Lùn* 傷寒論 is harmonization (*hé fǎ* 和法), which includes different strategies to harmonize Yīn and Yáng at the different layers of the body. This text subdivides Yīn and Yáng into six *jīng* 經 ("warps" or layers): Tàiyáng, Shàoyáng, Yángmíng, Tàiyīn, Shàoyīn, and Juéyīn. Each visceral system functions optimally when Yīn and Yáng are harmonized. In the Tàiyáng layer, we harmonize *yíng qì* 營氣 ("construction/provisioning" Qì) and *wèi qì* 衛氣 ("defense Qì"). *Yíng* is Yīn, *wèi* is Yáng, so that they compliment each other in regulating the *còulǐ* 腠理 ("interstices"), regulating sweating, and preventing exterior evils from permeating the interior, Yīn layer of the body where they can lodge in vital organs and tissues. In the Lung visceral system associated with Tàiyīn, the regulation of respiration (inhalation, exhalation) is also a form of regulating Yīn and Yáng. In the gastrointestinal system of the Stomach and Large Intestine associated with Yángmíng, peristalsis, the rhythmic regulation of expansion and contraction of the esophagus, stomach, and intestines is yet another expression of the movement of Yīn and Yáng. Loss of this rhythm can lead to constipation or diarrhea, heartburn, nausea or vomiting. In the Heart and Vessel visceral system of Shàoyīn, the rhythmic expansion and contraction of the heart and blood vessels, pumping blood and regulating its movement throughout the body is controlled by Yīn and Yáng. Loss of this rhythmic balance can lead to irregular heartbeat, palpitations, and blood pressure issues. The Shàoyáng layer, including the Gallbladder and Sānjiāo, is responsible for thermoregulation and correct dissemination and transformation of fluids in the body. Whether we use acupuncture and moxabustion or herbal medicine, Chinese medicine in all of these cases is seeking to regulate Yīn and Yáng in primal, practical levels that are rooted in a sophisticated cosmology.

Conclusion

To conclude this section, the Yellow Emperor once again emphasizes how the art of medicine is rooted in the resonances of Heaven and Earth in the human body through the medium of Yīn and Yáng. As we have encountered so often in this book, this final statement reiterates the central message of the *Great Treatise*, the resonance between Heaven, Humanity, and Earth. Through the language of two-fold complementarity in Yīn and Yáng, this book allows us to envision and elucidate the ideal state of harmony and balance with and between the infinite number of microcosms that make up the totality of the macrocosm. Once we grasp Yīn and Yáng, we can hone our senses to detect the slightest signs of imbalance and refine our skills at restoring the ideal dynamic equilibrium with elegant subtlety and the least effort necessary. Thereby we too can perfect the art of *zhì* 治, whether it means dredging continents to create arable land, ruling a state, or treating the human body. This art seems especially pertinent in our current world of global warming, nuclear proliferation, gene manipulation, and other human innovations with rapidly increasing potential to affect the macrocosmic balance to a far greater degree than ever imagined before. As such, it might behoove us to listen to the Yellow Emperor and his wise advisor Qí Bó as they contemplate the wisdom of the ancient sages at the dawn of Chinese civilization. The traces of their insights, as expressed in the Chinese medical and philosophical classics, offer this ideal of resonance with Yīn and Yáng as the crucial prism through which to view our role as humans in the great trinity of Heaven, Humanity, and Earth, whether we are trying to restore order in bodies, countries, or irrigation ditches. In the end, we are all One and we all hum together, from the humming bird above my head to the earthworm under my toe.

Reference List

I. Historical Sources – Alphabetical, by Pīnyīn Title

《大學》 *Dà Xué* (Great Learning). Anon., Hàn period.

《道德經》 *Dào Dé Jīng* (Classic of the Way and Virtue-Power). Láozi 老子, Warring States period.

《黃帝內經素問》 *Huáng Dì Nèi Jīng Sù Wèn* (Yellow Emperor's Inner Classic: Plain Questions). Anon., Hàn period. Commentary by Wáng Bīng 王冰, Táng period.

《黃帝內經素問集注》 *Huáng Dì Nèi Jīng Sù Wèn Jí Zhù* (Collected Commentaries on the Yellow Emperor's Inner Classic, Plain Questions). Zhāng Zhìcōng 張志聰, 1670.

《黃帝內經素問注証發微》 *Huáng Dì Nèi Jīng Sù Wèn Zhù Zhèng Fā Wéi* (The Yellow Emperor's Inner Classic, Plain Questions Annotated, Verified, and Explored in Detail). Mǎ Shì 馬蒔, 1586.

《黃帝素問直解》 *Huáng Dì Sù Wèn Zhí Jiě* (Straight Explanations of the *Huáng Dì Sù Wèn*). Gāo Shìzōng 高士宗, Qīng period.

《金匱要略》 *Jīn Guì Yào Lüè* (Essential Prescriptions from the Golden Cabinet). Zhāng Zhòngjǐng 張仲景, Eastern Hàn period.

《舊唐書》 *Jiù Táng Shū* (Old Book of the Táng). Compiled by Liú Xù et als., tenth century.

《類經》 *Lèi Jīng* (Categorized Classic). Zhāng Jièbīn 張介賓, 1624.

《禮記》 *Lǐ Jì* (Record of Rituals). Anon., Hàn period.

《內經知要》 *Nèi Jīng Zhī Yào* (Synopsis of the *Inner Classic*). Lǐ Zhōngzǐ 李中梓, 1642.

《神農本草經》 *Shén Nóng Běncǎo Jīng* (Divine Farmer's Classic of Materia Medica). Anon., Hàn period.

《聖濟總錄》 *Shèng Jì Zǒng Lù* (Comprehensive Record of the Sage's Rescue). Sòng Hūizōng 宋徽宗, 1112.

《史記》 *Shǐ Jì* (Records of the Historian). Sīmǎ Qiān 司馬遷, Hàn period.

《說文解字》 *Shuō Wén Jiě Zì* (Explaining Graphs and Elucidating Characters). Xǔ Shèn 許慎, 2nd c. CE.

《素問吳注》 *Sù Wèn Wú Zhù* (Commentary by Wú Kūn on the *Plain Questions*). Wú Kūn 吳崑, 1594.

《天下至道談》 *Tiān Xià Zhì Dào Tán* (Discussion of the Ultimate Dào Under Heaven). Anon., prior to 168 BCE.

《繫辭傳》 *Xì Cí Zhùan* (Commentary on the Appended Phrases). Anon., Hàn period.

《養性延命錄》 *Yǎng Xìng Yán Mìng Lù* (Record on Nurturing the Inner Nature and Extending Destiny). Táo Hóngjǐng 陶弘景, 6th century CE.

《易經》 *Yì Jīng* (Classic of Changes). Anon., Zhōu period.

II. Contemporary Sources – Alphabetical, by Author's Last Name

Bensky, Dan, and John O'Connor, *Acupunture: A Comprehensive Text, Shanghai College of Traditional Medicine* (Eastland Press, 1996).

Chace, Charles, and Miki Shima, *An Exposition on the Eight Extraordinary Vessels: Acupuncture, Alchemy, and Herbal Medicine* (Eastland Press, 2010).

Harper, Donald, *Early Chinese Medical Literature: The Mawangdui Medical Manuscripts* (Keegan Paul International, 1998).

Hsu, Elisabeth, "Outward Form (*xing* 形) and Inward Qi 氣: The 'Sentimental Body' in Early Chinese Medicine," *Early China* 32 (2009), pp. 103-24.

The Transmission of Chinese Medicine (Cambridge University Press, 1999).

Kimmerer, Robin Wall, *Braiding Sweetgrass: Indigenous Wisdom, Scientific Knowledge, and the Teachings of the Plants* (Milkweed Editions, 2013).

Kroll, Paul W., *A Student's Dictionary of Classical and Medieval Chinese* (Brill, 2015).

Maitri, Sandra, *The Enneagram of Passions and Virtues* (Penguin, 2009).

Ni, Maoshing, *The Yellow Emperor's Classic of Medicine: A New Translation of the Neijing Suwen with Commentary* (Shambhala, 1995).

Pearson, Margaret J., *The Original I Ching: An Authentic Translation of the Book of Changes Based on Recent Discoveries* (Tuttle Publishing, 2011).

Rochat de la Vallée, Elisabeth, *The Rhythm at the Heart of the World: Neijing Suwen Chapter 5* (Monkey Press, 2012).

Rosenberg, Z'ev, *Return to the Source: Han Dynasty Medical Classics in Clinical Practice* (Singing Dragon Press, forthcoming in 2017).

Roth, Harold D., *Original Tao: Inward Training (Nei-Yeh) and the Foundations of Taoist Mysticism* (Columbia University Press, 1999).

Unschuld, Paul U., *Was ist Medizin? Westliche und östliche Wege der Heilkunst* (Beck, 2003), published in English translation as *What is Medicine? Western and Eastern Approaches to Healing* (University of California, 2009).

Unschuld, Paul U., and Hermann Tessenow, *Huang Di Nei Jing Su Wen: An Annotated Translation of Huang Di's Inner Classic – Basic Questions* (University of California Press, 2011).

Veith, Ilza, *The Yellow Emperor's Classic of Internal Medicine* (University of California Press, 2002).

Wilms, Sabine, *The Divine Farmer's Classic of Materia Medica* (Happy Goat Productions, 2016).

Wiseman, Nigel, and Feng Ye, *A Practical Dictionary of Chinese Medicine* (Paradigm Publications, 1998).

Wiseman, Nigel, and Sabine Wilms, *Jīn Guì Yào Lüè: Essential Prescriptions of the Golden Cabinet* (Paradigm Publications, 2013).

Wu, Liansheng, and Qi Wu, *Yellow Emperor's Canon of Internal Medicine* (China Science and Technology Press, 2002).

CPSIA information can be obtained
at www.ICGtesting.com
Printed in the USA
FFOW03n0545170418
46224448-47568FF

9 781732 157101